# ASSESSING HEALTH AND HUMAN
# SERVICE NEEDS

# THE COMMUNITY PSYCHOLOGY SERIES

Sponsored by

the Division of Community Psychology of the
American Psychological Association

The Community Psychology Series has as its central purpose the building of philosophic, theoretical, scientific and empirical foundations for action research in the community and in its subsystems, and for education and training for such action research.

As a publication of the Division of Community Psychology, the series is particularly concerned with the development of community psychology as a subarea of psychology. In general, it emphasizes the application and integration of theories and findings from other areas of psychology, and in particular the development of community psychology methods, theories, and principles, as these stem from actual community research and practice.

# ASSESSING HEALTH AND HUMAN SERVICE NEEDS

*Concepts, Methods and Applications*

*Edited by*

**Roger A. Bell, Ed.D.**

*University of Louisville*
*Louisville, Kentucky*

**Martin Sundel, Ph.D.**

*University of Texas at Arlington*
*Arlington, Texas*

**Joseph F. Aponte, Ph.D.**

*University of Louisville*
*Louisville, Kentucky*

**Stanley A. Murrell, Ph.D.**

*University of Louisville*
*Louisville, Kentucky*

**Elizabeth Lin, M.S.**

*University of Louisville*
*Louisville, Kentucky*

**Volume VIII *Community Psychology Series***
Series Editor: Bernard Bloom, Ph.D.

Sponsored by Division of Community Psychology
American Psychological Association

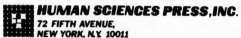

**HUMAN SCIENCES PRESS,INC.**
**72 FIFTH AVENUE,**
**NEW YORK, N.Y. 10011**

Copyright © 1983 by Human Sciences Press, Inc.
72 Fifth Avenue, New York, New York 10011

Printed in the United States of America
3456789   987654321

**Library of Congress Cataloging in Publication Data**
Main entry under title:

Assessing health and human service needs.

(The Community psychology series; v. 8)
Includes index.
1. Community health services—Evaluation.   2. Community mental health services—Evaluation.   3. Health status indicators.   4. Social indicators.   5. Health surveys.   I. Bell, Roger A.   II. Series.   [DNLM:
1. Health services research.   WA 525 A846]
RA427.A74        362.1        LC 81–20249
ISBN 0–89885–057–6                AACR2

ISSN  0731-0471

# CONTENTS

5

# CONTRIBUTORS

JOSEPH F. APONTE, Ph.D., Professor of Psychology, Director, Clinical Psychology Training Program, Department of Psychology, University of Louisville, Louisville, Kentucky

C. CLIFFORD ATTKISSON, Ph.D., Associate Professor of Psychology, Department of Psychiatry and the Langley Porter Institute, University of California, San Francisco, California

ROGER A. BELL, Ed.D., Professor, Department of Psychiatry and Behavioral Sciences and Family Medicine; Director, Psychiatric Medical Education, School of Medicine; Assistant Director for Health Systems, Systems Science Institute, University of Louisville, Louisville, Kentucky

BERNARD L. BLOOM, Ph.D., Professor of Psychology, Department of Psychology, University of Colorado, Boulder, Colorado

MARILYNN J. BOTTINO, M.A., Research Associate, Department of Psychiatry, University of California, San Francisco, California

9

ANTHONY BROSKOWSKI, Ph.D., Executive Director, Northside Community Mental Health Center, Inc.; Associate Professor, Department of Psychiatry, University of South Florida Medical School, Tampa, Florida

HAROLD W. DEMONE, JR., Ph.D., Dean, Graduate School of Social Work, Rutgers—The State University of New Jersey, New Brunswick, New Jersey

ANDRÉ L. DELBECQ, D.B.A., Dean, School of Business and Administration, University of Santa Clara, Santa Clara, California

BARBARA SNELL DOHRENWEND, Ph.D., Professor and Head, Division of Sociomedical Sciences, School of Public Health, Columbia University, New York

H. WARREN DUNHAM, Ph.D., Professor of Sociology, Emeritus, Wayne State University, Detroit, Michigan; Professor of Psychiatry (Sociology), State University of New York at Stony Brook, New York

DARLENE GOODHART, M.A., Research Associate, Department of Psychology, Arizona State University, Tempe, Arizona

MARCIA GUTTENTAG, Ph.D., formerly Richard Clarke Cabot Professor of Social Ethics, Harvard Graduate School of Education, Cambridge, Massachusetts

NANCY KOCHANOWICZ, M.A., Research Associate, Department of Psychology, Arizona State University, Tempe, Arizona

PAMELA M. LEONE, M.Ed., Doctoral Candidate, Community-Social Psychology Training Program, Department of Psychology, University of Louisville, Louisville, Kentucky

ELIZABETH LIN, M.S., Research Assistant, Department of Psychiatry and Behavioral Sciences, School of Medicine; Masters Candidate, System Sciences Institute, University of Louisville, Louisville, Kentucky

BENJAMIN LOCKE, M.S.P.H., Chief, Center for Epidemiological Studies, National Institute for Mental Health, Rockville, Maryland

STANLEY A. MURRELL, Ph.D., Professor of Psychology, Department of Psychology, University of Louisville; Director, Behavioral Science Applications, Urban Studies Center, University of Louisville, Louisville, Kentucky

LAWRENCE G. NEWBY, Ph.D., Assistant Professor (on leave), Department of Psychiatry and Behavioral Sciences, School of Medicine, University of Louisville; Associate Director of Kentucky Health Systems Agency-West, Inc., Louisville, Kentucky

TUAN D. NGUYEN, Ph.D., Research Psychologist and Coordinator of Program Evaluation, Program Evaluation Service, District V Mental Health Center and Department of Psychiatry, University of California, San Francisco, California

JANET SCHEFF, Ph.D., Associate Professor, Graduate School of Architecture and Planning, Division of Urban Planning, Columbia University, New York; Associate Professor, Graduate School of Planning, University of Puerto Rico, Rio Piedons, Puerto Rico

JOHN J. SCHWAB, M.D., Professor and Chairman, Department of Psychiatry and Behavioral Sciences, School of Medicine, University of Louisville, Louisville, Kentucky

MARTIN SUNDEL, Ph.D., Roy E. Dulak Professor, Graduate School of Social Work, University of Texas at Arlington, Arlington, Texas

DANIELLE TURNS, M.D., Associate Professor, Department of Psychiatry and Behavioral Sciences, School of Medicine, University of Louisville; Assistant Chief, Psychiatric Service, Veterans Administration Medical Center, Louisville, Kentucky

GEORGE J. WARHEIT, Ph.D., Professor of Sociology in Psychiatry, College of Medicine, University of Florida, Gainesville, Florida

ALEX ZAUTRA, Ph.D., Assistant Professor, Department of Psychology, Arizona State University, Tempe, Arizona

# FOREWORD

Once upon a time, in a country called the United States of America, people believed that there was so much wealth and natural resources that they could do whatever they wanted to regardless of the cost. The people believed that they could live any way they wanted without ever having to worry about tomorrow. . . .

So might a late twentieth century fable begin. For a period of about twenty years, starting at the close of World War II, most of us believed that for all practical purposes our resources were infinite. Since about 1965, that belief has been slowly crumbling and is being replaced by a growing conviction that our resources are limited and that prudence would dictate that we would be wise to think much more carefully about how those limited resources are expended. Out of this growing concern has come the modern field of need assessment: a field that seeks to provide an objective and rational approach to resource allocation.

This volume is comprehensive in its scope and has been painstakingly edited by a group of scholars long at the forefront of the field of need assessment. Not only are the major need assessment technologies critically examined, but the entire enterprise is viewed in a historical and conceptual perspective that will make the volume doubly useful. I am very pleased that the volume is part of the Community Psychology Series.

Bernard L. Bloom
General Editor

# PREFACE

The papers included in this volume were presented at two inter-disciplinary conferences on need assessment in health and human services. These conferences, held in March of 1976 and 1978, were sponsored by the Departments of Psychiatry and Behavioral Sciences, Psychology, and Family Medicine of the University of Louisville in cooperation with local and state human service agencies.

The major purpose of these conferences was to provide a medium for the exchange of information among health and mental health professionals and agency specialists interested in need assessment in the context of health and human service delivery systems. Accordingly, invitations were extended to individuals representing a variety of professions: behavioral scientists, health administrators, social workers, physicians, nurses, and information-processing specialists. The large number of participants indicates both the widespread interest in need assessment as well as the diverse and complex nature of the field.

The conferences were designed to provide a logical and systematic coverage of relevant concepts, methods, and issues. Topics ranged from the sociohistorical forces that preceded and

fostered need assessment to the current state of the art manifested in conceptual issues, methodologic considerations, and
the utilization of assessment data in program planning. Finally,
sessions were devoted to examining the research possibilities that
had been proposed in the conference presentations and sympo-
sia. Many of the resulting implications for the future of need
assessment are discussed in the concluding chapter of this
volume.

A number of persons helped to make these conferences and
this volume possible. The editors would particularly like to
acknowledge the assistance of Mary Beth McLellan and Joann
Buhl during the First National Conference and Dianne Bettin-
ger, Susie Brewer, Gussie Thompson, Neal Traven, and Cathy
West for their help in the Second Conference and in preparing,
editing, and proofing the final manuscript. Finally, to Penny Cox,
whose work was always accurate and timely and who coordinated
the final manuscript preparations, we would like to extend a very
special note of thanks.

In these acknowledgments, we wish also to pay special attention to Marcia Guttentag, a contributor to this book, who died on
November 8, 1977. Professor Guttentag was an internationally
recognized authority in program evaluation, a highly respected
researcher in social psychology, and a strong advocate for women
and the poor.

Professor Guttentag's work was highly regarded by her colleagues, as was evidenced by her election to the presidencies of
two different divisions in the American Psychological Association, being named to many editorial boards, presidential panels
and consultantships, and receiving frequent fellowships and
awards. She was an early influential leader in program evaluation, being instrumental on the Task Force on Evaluation in
Community Mental Health Training. Her most recent and
perhaps best known work was the *Handbook of Evaluation Research,*
a two-volume work she edited with E. L. Struening. Professor
Guttentag's untimely death has been a great loss to social psychology, program evaluation, and we believe, to need assessment.

The Editors

# INTRODUCTION

Need assessment activity has mushroomed in the last five years, pushed on by diverse social and professional forces. During this period, however, the development of concepts, methods, and application procedures has lagged behind, and, as a result, the field has not progressed in an even and systematic fashion. Furthermore, need assessment environments have included a variety of competing forces with quite differing purposes. These factors, combined with the multidisciplinary nature of need assessment endeavors, contribute to the diversity and the complex nature of the field. Although the field of need assessment holds great promise, it is still early in the process of development. This volume reflects the struggles and progress in its development and outlines its future prospects.

The basic activity of need assessment seems straightforward enough: a human service agency collects information about its potential "customers" and then uses that information to revise existing programs and develop new ones. The strong face-valid reasonableness of this basic idea is probably the single most important force for the rapid increase in need assessment activities.

However, need assessments are not done in a vacuum. They are conceived of and performed in a vortex of competing pushes and pulls from different groups with different values. Such pressures derive from a practical fact: need assessments have the potential to determine who gets what amount of which resources. These competing constituencies vary with the local situation, but they typically include the following:

*Behavioral scientists* who are interested in theory construction and hypothesis building. They consequently value need assessment data as ends as much as means and are concerned about protecting the integrity of those data.

*Elected officials* who value the potential of need assessments for making programs more visibly responsive to voters and for wresting some control over programs from bureaucrats and professionals.

*Funding agencies,* which are typically ambivalent toward need assessments. They may fear possible reductions in their bureaucratic discretionary power in resource allocation, and yet, at the same time, value the potential for increasing documentation and accountability from service agencies, and the consequent leverage for program change.

*Service agencies,* which may also be ambivalent. On the one hand, they may resent the implicit criticism of their professional judgment inherent in need assessment as well as fear imposition of program changes from funding sources. On the other hand, they may favor a more rational basis for resource allocation decisions and hope for new program opportunities on the basis of assessment data.

*Service recipients* who, ironically, are typically the least directly involved. They remain a potential pressure however, and as respondents in need assessments they are usually appreciative of the opportunity for input to the data-gathering and planning process.

Through the early phases of need assessment development, these constituencies have had differing purposes and have applied pressures for different kinds of assessments. *Thus, a reality of need assessments is that they take place not in laboratories but in arenas that are ultimately political.*

## HISTORICAL FORCES

None of the components of need assessment are unique to the field. Its present separate identity derives from the particular linkage of these borrowed parts at a propitious time under a newly clarified purpose. There have been a number of influences in both the professional and societal cultures that have helped forge this linkage and have thus accelerated the development of need assessment techniques and concepts.

World War II served as the necessity that mothered many inventions. One of these was the extremely rapid development of *computer technology* that allowed for quantification on a much grander scale than had earlier been possible. Starkly representative of this new influence was the career of Robert McNamara who brought his war experience in operations research to the peacetime industry of making Ford automobiles. With this application, operations research gained the stamp of real practical value and was subsequently accepted into government when McNamara became Secretary of Defense in the Kennedy administration. The rationalistic emphasis in this administration, combined with the quantification emphasis of operations research, led to a new formula: resource decisions would be made strictly on the basis of quantitative evidence. This general trend, which might be called the *data-for-decisions movement,* persisted beyond Kennedy's administration, McNamara's tenure, or military hardware decisions to affect government decisions about resource allocation. Today we take it for granted that such politically sensitive decisions as federal funds for public education or unemployment aid to cities are determined largely by quantitative data.

It is not surprising, therefore, that the data-for-decisions movement eventually spread from decisions about military hardware to the so-called soft social and health services that had heretofore been dominated by professional expertise. By the time it reached them, however, this technological movement had been joined by two demands: one for greater responsiveness followed by the second for increased accountability.

The call for greater responsiveness perhaps became articulated first in the antipoverty programs in the mid-1960s. Recipients demanded more control over the programs designed ostensibly to assist them out of poverty. Soon, individuals in other sectors began to raise similar questions about control. Expressed in various ways, about different issues, the essence of their complaint was that citizens had no voice in decisions that subsequently affect them. Some behavioral scientists and service professionals joined in this criticism. And, indeed, the thrust of this complaint became the foundation for at least one new field, community psychology, and has continued to be a central value for it and other behavioral science areas.

Eventually, legislation was generated that required some form of citizen participation before certain kinds of resource decisions were made. At first, these decisions were primarily with respect to the physical environment, for example, for community development funds or for environmental changes that required "impact" statements. However, the responsiveness ideology soon reached the health and human service fields, where the terminology referred to "health status" and "need assessment," terms that went largely undefined in the press for implementation.

To be responsive required that programs be oriented more toward the priorities of the service recipients and less toward those of the providers. The second force, that of accountability, required that programs be justified to funding agencies on more evidence than simply professional or clinical judgments of service providers.

"Accountability" is in fashion at the time of this writing, having been reinforced by the "Proposition 13" ideology that tax money not be wasted and that bureaucracies demonstrate the effectiveness of their programs. However, this is a relatively new emphasis. It was not until the mid-1960s that it was first articulated by elected officials, who ostensibly were concerned about the waste in antipoverty programs. The initial questioning about the effectiveness of these specific programs led to increased evaluation and assessment activities. This concern for accountability eventually spread beyond antipoverty efforts to encompass the health and human service fields.

These two influences represent quite different values: responsiveness is concerned that recipients not be ill served, while accountability is concerned that the tax money of government not be misused. Both, however, added to the impetus for doing assessments of need.

While all three forces—the data-for-decisions movement and the demands for accountability and responsiveness—provided the energy for mobilizing action, they did not enlighten the process. They pushed but did not steer. There was little real understanding of program design requirements or of the types of management decisions faced by service agencies. The motivations and training of service professionals were typically either disregarded or denigrated. Consequently, the nature of the program task and the organizational environment were rarely considered in the rush to implement need assessments.

In the early stages, under the mounting pressure for concrete results, the outlines of what a need assessment "should be" slowly developed. The assessment process needed to provide data that were: (1) quantitative; (2) "uncontaminated" by service agency personnel to insure objectivity; (3) from or about the catchment population to insure program relevance to recipients; and (4) able to provide documentation to justify resource allocation decisions. These rudimentary criteria primarily reflected the interests of three constituencies: elected officials, funding agencies, and recipients. Left out were the concerns of the behavioral scientists, the people who were to *collect* the data, and the service agency groups, the people who were to *use* the data in their programs.

As versions of this outline began to appear in legislation and in federal program regulations, and as service agencies were increasingly required to conduct assessments following such guidelines, the previously neglected question of "how" came to the fore. Since the quantitative emphasis was strong, service agencies tried to turn to the behavioral sciences. One dilemma arose immediately, which discipline to turn to? There was no academic field of need assessment. There was no single discipline that had developed a systematic set of concepts, principles, or methods tailored in particular for need assessment. Thus, assessments were conducted before a coherent foundation of clear definitions and appropriate methods could be established.

Given these circumstances, it was perhaps inevitable that those behavioral scientists who found themselves doing need assessments borrowed from a wide spectrum of fields to accomplish their purposes. With the pressure for fast compliance, the first emphasis was on methods. From *epidemiology* came a major research tool, the field survey, along with the recognition of the advantages and disadvantages of using case records. The use of in-depth interviews was borrowed from the *clinical areas* and applied to individuals or "key informants" in the community who were expected to be especially knowledgeable about the needs in question. From *economics* was borrowed the idea of using indicators, but for need assessment these were social rather than economic in nature. Demographic variables such as marital status, sex, age, etc. were assumed to reflect health and social need, at least indirectly and moreover were easily available from the U.S. Census. From *community organization* came the idea of community forums and the techniques to facilitate such grass roots meetings among possible program recipients. And, in addition, techniques from the various behavioral or social sciences of epidemiology, sociology, psychology, psychiatry, education, anthropology, and political science were expediently rather than systematically applied: a concept here, a technique there, a finding somewhere else.

The diversity of terms and orientations inevitable from such multidisciplinary efforts was increased further by the wide variation in local conditions. As numerous individual need assessments were tailored for their own particular need-types, populations, or funding sources, they contributed to a profusion of terms, measures, methods, and application procedures. Moreover, they were all being done more or less simultaneously, rather than in an orderly stepwise progression, making it difficult for assessors to learn from one another's mistakes. This volume attempts through its reporting of the cumulative experience of need assessors over the past several years to contribute an improved sense of directionality to the field.

## PRESENT STAGE OF DEVELOPMENT

Where does need assessment stand today? What has been learned from all this need assessment activity? How should the performance of need assessment to date be judged? Slowly, the broad range of experiences is being sifted and certain directions are becoming evident, reflected in the current consensus, in lessons that have been learned, and in the criticisms of need assessment.

One current opinion is that the concept of "need" requires increased clarity. Recent work, reported in this volume, aimed at comparing the appropriateness as well as the efficacy of different approaches to measuring "need" addresses this issue.

Another current opinion is that different levels of need must be clearly distinguished. The preferences expressed in this volume are for going beyond the individual level to include the family, organization, and community.

In early efforts, a single method applied to a limited subpopulation could legitimately serve as a need assessment. The consensus has since developed, through haphazard trial and error, that the combined use of several different methods is highly desirable. Such a convergent approach has the potential to provide more comprehensive and accurate data than any single approach.

These early experiences also revealed that need assessors who did not understand an agency's ideology and who were not familiar with its programs might well provide data that were irrelevant from the agency's perspective and therefore unlikely to be used. Thus, the value of a close working relationship between the data collectors and data users at all stages has begun to be accepted, and procedures have been suggested to aid that linkage.

Related to this recognition, need assessors have been gradually awakening to the fact that the clinical orientation of most health and human service agencies made them unprepared for and unreceptive to the implications of need assessments: first, agencies were oriented to present demand for services, not to long-term planning; and second, agencies were oriented to individual patients, not to populations. In short, it is now recognized that the ideology of need assessment has not matched the ideology of service agencies that are expected to use the resulting data.

It has also been true that as experiences with need assessments have increased, so have the criticisms. Considering the initial handicaps of need assessments—the competing constituencies, the lack of a systematic conceputal or methodologic foundation, the unclear connections between data and programs, and the ambivalence of service agencies—it was perhaps inevitable that early performances were not particularly impressive. It was also probably inevitable that the practice of need assessment received numerous criticisms from different sources. While many of these criticisms have some basis, they need to be placed in perspective.

The particulars of these criticisms have varied according to which constituency the critic belonged to, but four stand out as perhaps being the most general and most frequent: (1) assessment data often do not yield new information, and service providers already know about the needs; (2) the term *need* is often ill-defined and often not clearly distinguished from "want"; (3) the validity and reliability of need measures have not been established; and (4) after being collected, assessment data are often not used in program decisions. Each of these criticisms is expressed and addressed in the chapters that follow.

First with respect to "new" information, needs are ubiquitous in the human experience, are expressed constantly, and take different forms. It is not realistic to expect that the methods of need assessments will invariably discover previously unknown needs! It *is* realistic, however, to expect need assessments to measure need comprehensively and systematically, and to provide an *ordering* of needs. It is also not realistic to expect need assessments to provide information that service professionals admit is new to them. In the first place, to do so would not reflect well on their competence, but in any case service professionals spend their entire careers hearing about the various and multiple needs of individual clients; what they do not have is *systematic* and *ordered* information about the needs of a catchment *population* that need assessments can realistically provide. With *this* kind of information, it is possible for program managers to reallocate resources, to develop or refine programs for those problems with the highest priorities, or for those at-risk populations that have the greatest relative need.

With respect to the need to define concepts and to establish the reliability and validity of measures, concepts and measure definitely need to be improved, but it is unrealistic to expect a highly refined technology overnight. No discipline has ever sprung into being with concepts fully explicated or value and reliable measure already established. These refinements develop with experience, criticism, testing, refinement, and further testing; it is an ongoing process, we are at its beginning, and this volume reflects the necessary criticisms and attempted refinements toward further development. But, it is certainly true that we must be especially concerned about the accuracy and meaning of need assessment data. It is also realistic to expect that stronger efforts be made to evaluate the validity and responsiveness of measures used in need assessments.

With respect to the program use of need assessment data, it seems clear that to expect such data to have exclusive or immediate effects on program decisions is to ignore powerful organizational and institutional realities. Even the best assessment data possible would remain only one of several competing information inputs to organizational decisions. Moreover, the organizational and institutional structures are typically very strongly supportive of existing programs. It is perhaps most realistic at this stage to view need assessment data as making their most valuable contributions to documentation and to planning, not to immediate program change. Application of any sort will require time for service providers to become familiar and comfortable with the data. In general, data usage will require greater program sophistication by the data collectors and greater data sophistication by the service agencies, and these competencies are slowly developing.

## PROSPECTS

Given the number of criticisms and the tumultuous early circumstances of need assessments, it is a strong testimonial to the power of their face-valid purpose and the supporting cultural trends that they have not only survived but increased in number in the past five years. This fact argues for the clear relevance of need assessment for present day priorities. But what are the prospects for the future?

In evaluating the past performance and, more importantly at this stage, estimating the promise of need assessment, a number of factors must be considered. First, the success of need assessment is highly dependent upon the quality and nature of program management. Some of the application failures of need assessment have been due, not to the irrelevance of the data, but to inadequate levels of program conceptualization and operation. For need assessment to become increasingly valuable, there must be parallel improvements in program management, for example, better program design, more sophisticated budgeting techniques, better program evaluation and management information systems. Hopefully, need assessment and program management will improve and develop in an integrated manner.

A second question to consider is the most effective scale for need assessment. The bulk of assessments done to date have been small, by single agencies, and have typically been one-shot efforts. Since need assessment is primarily a *population* tool, it may turn out that its greatest utility is for large populations such as at the state or regional levels. And, if the planning function comes to be clearly paramount, need assessments that are done repeatedly at regular intervals over long periods of time may be used to indicate trends and to forecast future needs.

A third factor, and related to the question above, is the comprehensiveness of the needs assessed. While most efforts to date have assessed only one type of need at a time (for example, mental health need, health need), need assessments may be particularly valuable for assessing the wide range of needs as experienced by recipients, not only mental health but also housing, employment, and social activities, for example. This would then allow planners to examine a wide spectrum of needs in a systematic, comparative fashion. However, this value would probably depend on being at regional or state level of planning.

At this time, two very different future directions seem possible. Need assessment may turn out to be a narrow and temporary technology; a fad activity that was fostered by a *Zeitgeist* but then allowed to flounder by behavioral science, service agencies, and funding agencies. Or, need assessment may become part of a planning science that eventually comes to have a powerful influence on institutional, agency, and program development. The development of such influence will require the continuation of the conceptual, methodologic, and program application developments reported in this volume. It will also require fertile management environments. It may be facilitated by increases in the scale, duration, and comprehensiveness of need assessments in the future.

To some degree, the ultimate fate of need assessment lies with future societal events and the trends in the social and professional cultures. But, beyond such external influences, the energy, intelligence, and thoughtfulness of need assessors, both behavioral scientists and agency managers, in guiding the development of need assessment in the next five years will be crucial. It is our hope that this volume will make a useful contribution to that continuing development.

Stanley A. Murrell<br>
Joseph F. Aponte<br>
Elizabeth Lin

Part I

# ORIENTATION TO NEED ASSESSMENT

## INTRODUCTION

The initial section of this volume provides a general orientation to assessing health and human service needs. Schwab indentifies several sociohistorical forces at work today that have led to the demand for need assessment. He traces these demands back to the case register work, started in 1775, that provided human service workers with the first tools to begin to analyze the distribution of illness in the general population.

These initial efforts developed in the area of epidemiology, that is, the measurement of illness in the general population, and were the stepping stones into the area of need assessment, which attempts the measurement of identified need in a community context. The early work of Dunham, the second author in this section, on mental disorder in urban areas provides an example of ways to estimate needs in the general population.

In addition to the methodologic strategies that have developed, there are other sociohistorical forces, such as the role of the federal government in requiring that programs and resource allocation be tied to identified need. Locke discusses the relationship of epidemiology and need assessment to some of the directions that he and his colleagues at the federal level are taking. Locke also makes a useful distinction between need assessment and epidemiologic methods.

Thus, some of the political, social, and historical forces that serve as the basis and motivation for need assessment are identified in this first section. This orientation provides a background for the conceptual and theoretical issues, methodologic aspects, and role of program planning in need assessment to be discussed in the subsequent sections of this book.

*Chapter 1*

# IDENTIFYING AND ASSESSING NEEDS

## A Synergism of Social Forces

*John J. Schwab*

The zeal of the philanthropist was awakened to the pitiable situation of lunatics; and the attention of the learned was directed to a malady, evidently but little understood.

George Man Burrows, 1820[1]

Needs are basic to the human condition. Simply, yet profoundly, Masserman[2] has described man's three primordial Ur needs: (1) the biologic requisites for survival: air, water, food, and shelter; (2) the interpersonal needs for companionship and affection essential for a sense of identity, emotional expression, and a meaningful existence; and (3) the spiritual yearnings for a faith or a metaphysic that gives a transcendent meaning to life. When basic needs are not fulfilled because of personal inadequacies (biologic as well as social) or because of frustration, conflict, and deprivation, mental illness often results.

But persons defined as mentally ill are only one segment of

31

the group requiring mental health care. Others are those with psychic distress and interpersonal and social problems stemming from: (1) lack of milieu reliability, dependable relationships, and cultural sustenance; (2) ill-defined boundaries and an inadequate reality orientation resulting in difficulties with daily tasks and routines; (3) a dearth of opportunities for personal fulfillment, freedom of choice, and role continuity; and (4) a paucity of performance rewards and group affirmation.[3]

An assessment of needs for health and human service, therefore, will uncover evidence of overlapping bodily, interpersonal, and spiritual distress. Mental disorders and the needs for mental health care seldom appear as isolated disturbances. They involve persons, not just phenomena, and their manifestations affect groups and communities, not just individuals. As Francis Bacon[4] wrote more than 300 years ago:

> Human philosophy, or humanity, hath two parts: the one considereth man segregate or distributively: the other, congregate or in society.

For two centuries, since the British Parliament's Act to regulate asylums established a Case Register in 1775,[5] physicians and social scientists have been attempting to identify persons with mental disorders and estimate their number. Usually, these scientific endeavors sprang from two sources: (1) concern about the availability of services and quality of care provided the mentally ill, and (2) investigators' hopes that they could ascertain individual, familial, and social factors associated with mental illness, and that greater knowledge about these factors would reduce human suffering.

Assessment of mental health needs in Western society began with Richard Powell's[5] analysis of the data in the Case Register started in 1775. In 1810, he reported to the Royal College of Physicians that insanity had increased between the years 1775 to 1809. But Powell noted that the results of his study were questionable because both case reporting and the Census figures were inaccurate. Since Powell's initial endeavor, such rates-under-treatment studies have been conducted many times in an attempt to measure the extent of mental illness although they are subject to the limitations noted by Powell,[5] Burrows,[1] and Esquirol[6] in the early decades of the nineteenth century. Furthermore, the institutionalized, and even those receiving any type of treatment, are selected groups—selected by self, by others, or by the community for care or incarceration—and thus are not representative of the general population. Also, they reflect a society's labeling process and its seeming need to extrude a certain segment of its population. Therefore, the data derived from rates-under-treatment studies cannot be accepted as accurate estimates of the need for mental health care.

Some of the rates-under-treatment studies, however, have made significant contributions to our knowledge about mental illness and society. In the 1820s Esquirol[6] showed that observed increases in the number of mentally ill in France occurred only where there were improved facilities and services. More than a century later, in the 1930s, Faris and Dunham[7] found that differential rates of admissions to mental hospitals in urban areas could be associated with distinctive ecologic patterns. About the same time, Roth and Luton's[8] comparisons of admission rates to hospitals with examinations of the general population in Williamson County, Tennessee, revealed the deficiencies of the health delivery system; almost 50 percent of those with psychoses had not received treatment. And Hollingshead and Redlich's[9] intensive New Haven study in the 1950s showed that the type of care received by patients varied according to their social class status.

In addition to the knowledge gleaned about the relationships between social processes and mental illness, these major studies have exposed the discrepancies between mental health needs and the availability of treatment services.

Mental illness is one of our foremost public health problems. The toll in human suffering and even in increased mortality is alarming. In 1972 Rosenthal[10] reported to the National Academy of Sciences that there were 1.75 million potential schizophrenics at large and another 500,000 were in hospitals. About 9 million Americans have serious drinking problems. In April 1978, the President's Commission on Mental Health reported that "25 percent of all Americans (about 55 million people) suffer from mental problems and that 15 percent need some form of mental health services."[11] Data published in 1975 indicated that of the 15 million Americans suffering with depression, only 1.5 million received treatment. And the number of suicides, probably 50,000, matched the number who died from diabetes or leukemia.[12]

Other studies reveal that mental illness is associated, directly or indirectly, with increased mortality. Levine and Levine[13] report that studies using the Monroe County Register (New York) indicate that the excess death risk between 1960 and 1966 for persons with common mental illnesses was almost twice that of comparable groups without diagnosed mental disorders. A study of U.S. Army veterans was confirmatory; compared to controls, those discharged with a diagnosis of psychoneurosis had an excess death rate of 21 percent.

Levine and Levine[13] estimate that the cost in dollars of mental illness in 1971 was $25 billion. Almost all of the direct cost, $11 billion, was spent for health programs. This was "13.2 percent of all health expenditures in the nation that year." The indirect costs were more than $14 billion. But they believe that these are conservative figures, and that the total cost is closer to $50 billion than to the $25 billion they computed.

Just the magnitude of the cost in human suffering, impairments, mortality, and dollars is probably sufficient reason for conducting systematic studies of needs for mental health services. But other compelling forces, social and historical, have converged to give the topic of need assessment in health and human services timeliness as well as importance. Many of the forebodings expressed by philosophers and social historians have appeared as the harsh realities of the twentieth century. Both Adam Smith[14] and Nietzche[15] feared that self-interest would emerge as a dominant disintegrating characteristic of modern life. Durkheim[16] and later Merton[17] depicted the consequences of anomic confusion, insecurity, and normlessness. And, early in this century, Max Weber[18] wondered whether "specialists without spirit, sensualists without heart" would live in this "cage in the future."

Two world wars, many other small wars, the Great Depression, widespread migration, displacement of peoples, and threat of overpopulation have been the tragedies of our era. Proliferative technology and the rapid rate of social change have been accompanied by alterations in society's forms and institutions.

Skepticism about our institutions' capabilities and disillusionment with many governmental programs have led to apathy, protests for reform, and demands for probity. We are now in the "age of accountability."[19] Assessment of needs for mental health services, therefore, is critically necessary in order to design programs that will meet the challenges of the age and contribute to the vitality as well as to the health of our society.

Despite awareness of the inadequacies of the health delivery system and despite the emergence of the community mental health movement, very few systematic investigations of needs have been conducted. How to do it—efficiently and accurately— is a problem about which there is some disagreement.

We have several methods for assessing needs for services. The first assessment in the United States utilized the key informant approach. In Connecticut in 1812,[20] reports from physicians and officials throughout the state showed that there were 1,000 mentally ill persons, 1 of every 262 inhabitants. Amariah Brigham, the first editor of *The American Journal of Psychiatry*, noted that this estimate was thought to be too low. Another, more vivid, historical study was carried out in 1819 by Andrew Halliday[21] who polled the 900 Parishes in Scotland, obtained returns from 800, and reported that the total number of mentally ill was 3,700 in contrast to the 658 found in the public records. Moreover, of the 3,700, 1,861, not 658, were actually confined while the rest were wandering at large and begging.

The key informant approach to need assessment has only limited and variable utility in modern America; geographic mobility, expanding suburbs, and ghettoization allow for anonymity. Key informants probably can supply more significant information about special types of programs for their communities than identification or enumeration of those needing care.

The social indicators approach, relying on Census data and public records, is widely utilized by Community Mental Health Centers to assess needs for services. Such assessments are based on inferences that income levels, crime rates, housing conditions, and other measures of the quality of life are associated with certain frequencies of mental disorders and/or mental health needs. This approach provides little direct evidence about the numbers needing mental health care and the types of care required. But its development, only in the last few decades, and its increasing use reflects our society's concern with the quality of the social environment and its relationship to health and social needs. The epidemiologic method, involving interviews with or examinations of systematically selected samples of the general population, has greater scientific merit. Investigators employing this approach, however, are handicapped by conceptual and methodologic difficulties: problems with the definition of mental health or illness, case finding, response bias, and others. In the United States, major epidemiologic assessments have shown that frighteningly high percentages of the general population suffer from the impairments associated with mental illness. For example, in the Midtown Manhattan Study[22] in the 1950s, 23.4 percent of a random sample were rated impaired and, recently, in the 20-year follow-up, Srole[23] reports that 18.4 percent are impaired. The sheer magnitude of these percentages can paralyze program developers, who fear that their limited material and human resources are insufficient to meet the need. Nevertheless, well-designed studies, such as those carried out by Essen-Möller[24] and Hagnell[25] in Lundby, Sweden, have successfully identified high-risk persons and groups, measured both the incidence and prevalence of mental disorder in the community, and increased our knowledge about some relationships between social processes and mental illness.

Despite their limitations, epidemiologic assessments of needs for mental health services have utility. Systematic assessments identify persons and groups needing care and reveal variable types of needs. Thus, the information enables program planners to design services tailored to meet these needs and to improve our mental health delivery systems. Furthermore Bloom[26] emphasizes that epidemiology is the "basic science of preventive action."

Epidemiologic assessments, moreover, supply the necessary baseline data for evaluation, now rightfully demanded by our society in this "age of accountability." Evaluation proceeds through stages which compare the need for services with their utilization. Such evaluations should be sufficiently comprehensive to include measurement and scrutiny of outcomes and costs.

Elsewhere, I have mentioned that evaluation research is a necessary scientific endeavor that is pragmatic, humanistic, and teleologic. It is pragmatic in that it looks at phenomena in terms of antecedent conditions and results and emphasizes their utility.

It is humanistic in that it deals with major societal problems, for example, mental illness and deviance, and also with individuals' dilemmas. It is teleologic in that it regards phenomena not solely as mechanistic forces and events, but also as processes moving toward goals; thus, it considers consequences as well as techniques.[19]

Throughout this chapter I have alluded to the synergy of forces—humanitarian concerns, scientific pursuits, and compelling historical and social processes—that have culminated in our current interest in the assessment of needs for mental health care. To those forces we should add governmental and other planners' mandates to allocate human and material resources wisely and prudently, the necessity for program directors to develop efficient and effective services, and mental health workers' aspirations to offer care and succor to human beings with their variable needs and frailties.

Assessing needs for mental health services requires courage and commitment as well as knowledge and skills. How to meet the plethora of needs and respond to the catalogue of human misery that may be revealed by the assessment might raise questions about the ordering of our society's priorities and entail, in Thomas Kuhn's words, a "restructuring of commitments."[27]

In this report we should recall that Sigmund Freud, many years ago in 1919, in the "Turnings of the Ways in Psycho-Analytic Therapy,"[28] said that someday:

> the conscience of the community will awake and admonish it that the poor man has just as much right to help for his mind as he now has to the surgeon's means of saving life; and that the neuroses menace the health of a people no less than tuberculosis, and can be left as little as the latter to the feeble handling of individuals.

## NOTES

1. Burrows, G. M. *Is insanity an increasing malady? An inquiry into certain errors relative to insanity; and their consequences; physical, moral and civil.* London: Thomas and George Underwood, 1820.
2. Masserman, J. H. *The practice of dynamic psychiatry.* Philadelphia: Saunders, 1955.

3.  *The community worker: A response to human need.* Group for the Advancement of Psychiatry, Vol. IX, Report No. 91, 1974.

4.  Bacon, F., cited in Hill, D. The bridge between neurology and psychiatry. *The Lancet,* 1975, *1,* 509–517.

5.  Powell, R. Observations upon the comparative prevalance of insanity at different periods. In *Medical transactions.* London: Longman, 1813.

6.  Esquirol, J. E. A treatise on insanity (trans. 1845). In C. E. Goshen (Ed.), *Documentary history of psychiatry.* New York: Philosophical Library, 1967.

7.  Faris, R. E. L., & Dunham, H. W. *Mental disorders in urban areas: An ecological study of schizophrenia and other psychoses.* New York: Hafner, 1961.

8.  Roth, W. F., & Luton, F. H. The mental health program in Tennessee I. Description of the original study program; II. Statistical report of a psychiatric survey in a rural county. *The American Journal of Psychiatry,* 1943, *99*(9), 662–675.

9.  Hollingshead, A. B., & Redlich, R. C. *Social class and mental illness.* New York: John Wiley & Sons, Inc., 1958.

10. Rosenthal, D. *The Gainesville Sun,* Monday, April 24, 1972, p. 3-A.

11. *President's Commission on Mental Health Report.* Louisville Courier-Journal, 28 April 1978, A3.

12. Annual Meeting, National Association for Mental Health, Washington, D.C., 1975.

13. Levine, D. S., & Levine, D. R. *The cost of mental illness—1971.* National Institute of Mental Health, DHEW Publication No. (ADM) 76–265, Superintendent of Documents, Washington, D.C.: U.S. Government Printing Office, 1975.

14. Smith, A. *An inquiry into the nature and causes of the wealth of nations.* London: George Bell & Sons, 1892.

15. Morgan, G. A. *What Nietzche means.* New York: Harper Torchbooks (Harper & Row Publishers, Inc.), 1965.

16. Durkheim, E. *Suicide: A study in sociology.* Glencoe, Ill.: The Free Press, 1951.

17. Martindale, D. A. *The nature and types of sociological theory.* Boston: Houghton Mifflin, 1960.

18.  Weber, M. *The Protestant ethic and the spirit of capitalism.* New York: Scribner, 1958.

19.  Schwab, J. J. *Evaluation research and the community mental health movement.* Proceedings of the Florida Mental Health Evaluation Consortium. Tampa, Florida, May 29, 1974.

20.  Hunter, R., & MacAlpine, I. *Three hundred years of psychiatry.* New York: Oxford University Press, 1963, pp. 821–825.

21.  Halliday, A. *A general view of the present state of lunatics, and lunatic asylums, in Great Britain and Ireland, and in some other kingdoms.* London: Thomas and George Underwood, 1828.

22.  Langner, T., & Michael, S. T. *The Midtown Manhattan study: Life, stress and mental health.* New York: Crowell-Collier, 1963.

23.  Srole, L. Measurement and classification in the sociopsychiatric epidemiology: Midtown Manhattan study (1954) and Midtown Manhattan restudy (1974). *Journal of Health and Social Behavior,* January 1976.

24.  Essen-Möller, E. *Individual traits and morbidity in a Swedish rural population.* Copenhagen: Ejnar Munksgaard, 1956.

25.  Hagnell, O. *A prospective study of the incidence of mental disorder.* Lund, Sweden: Scandinavian University Books, 1966.

26.  Bloom, B. L. Strategies for the prevention of mental disorders. In G. Rosenblum (Ed.), *Issues in community psychiatry and preventive mental health.* New York: Behavioral Publications, 1971.

27.  Kuhn, T. *Structure of scientific revolutions.* Chicago: University of Chicago Press, 1962.

28.  Freud, S. The turnings of the ways. In E. Jones (Ed.), *Collected papers* (Vol. 2). The International Psycho-Analytical Library No. 8. New York: Basic Books, 1959.

*Chapter 2*

# THE EPIDEMIOLOGIC STUDY OF MENTAL ILLNESS

## Its Value for Need Assessment

## *H. Warren Dunham*

In this chapter I propose to examine epidemiologic studies of mental disorder as instruments for need assessment. I think I can achieve this objective by analyzing the impact of the past 50 years upon my own 1930 ecologic study.[1] In fact, this early study provided a basis, if the question had been asked then, for determining the need for psychiatric services in the Chicago metropolitan area.

Epidemiologic studies through measures such as age and sex specific rates provide a firm foundation not only for determining the number of people in a given catchment area with a specific disease (prevalence count), but also the number of new cases that develop within the course of a year (incidence count). Such figures can also be projected in relation to the population for at least a decade.

It is well recognized that epidemiologic studies of mental disease include only those persons who are defined by self or others as mentally ill. Thus, those who are sick but not defined as such go unrecognized. However, it is the former group that always is detected regardless of the available services thus providing a firm basis for the determination of minimal needs. Persons in the latter group tend to surface through encouragement by media propaganda, a sharp increase in psychiatric facilities available, and/or a legal tightening of conformity norms in the community.

Here, the terrain is quite murky, and if labeling theory has any significance, it is right here. That is, with our zest to help and our eagerness to heal, we often label persons as sick who are just different or have life styles that differ markedly from our own. Even so, no doubt some in this category do need psychiatric treatment provided they can be detected. It may never be possible to estimate the true percentage of undetected cases. The reason, I suspect, is because this percentage varies with time and place due to the radical changes in social organization and cultural patterns. This group of cases, when estimated and added to the first group, would provide some notion of the maximum in mental health needs for a given catchment area. One law seems to hold—an increase in psychiatric facilities means an increase in the number of persons using their services.

Consequently, my purpose here with respect to our pioneer epidemiologic study is not only to view its value at the time as a need assessment instrument but also to point to the continued reinterpretation of its positive findings produced by the social changes of the past 50 years.

While it may seem like "sour grapes" to take a backward glance and refer to the "good old days," I think a case can be made for the fact that at the time of our study, there was more stability to our general community life when compared to our communities today. Further, it seems to me that we were most positive about the definitions and labels that were bandied about whether we attached them to persons or to social structures. We had faith about what we knew, and we confidently thought that continual research would clear up those areas where our knowledge was lacking.

The straightforwardness of our thinking with respect to definitions is seen in our views about mental illness. When persons did become mentally ill, they were committed to a public mental hospital or, if from affluent families, placed in a private sanitarium. While some of the people outside these institutions might be regarded as mentally ill, little thought was given to them until they were so defined by family members, neighbors, employers, agency officials, or the police.[2]

In this connection, it is of interest to note the three criticisms by psychiatrists of our early effort to portray the distribution of selected psychoses in the community. First, the rates were held to be unreliable because they did not take into account the cases that never came to the attention of agency or government officials. One notes that this is a criticism that plagues these studies today.[3] My answer, at the time, was that the undetected cases in the community would eventually be committed or admitted voluntarily to a mental hospital. This was the recognition of what I later termed "the gap," that is, the time between initial symptom development and admission to a psychiatric facility. This gap has been shown to vary with socioeconomic level.[4]

A second criticism was that the diagnoses were unreliable. Therefore, there was little point in studying the distribution of rate patterns of specific psychoses. This resulted from two factors, namely, lack of knowledge about etiology and the differing psychiatric orientations found in training programs. In answer, I noted that while the psychiatrists emphasized the unreliability of the diagnoses in the clinical situation, they often defended the diagnosis that they had attached to the patient.

A third criticism contended that the rates pattern was misleading because it represented the residential mobility of the mentally sick rather than their community of origin. This is the well known "drift" hypothesis.[5] However, we were sociologists and had conducted the study from the perspective of human ecology, a theoretical position which motivated many studies at the University of Chicago in those days. As sociologists, we had not paid sufficient attention to the field of epidemiology, which had been successful in getting at the etiologic factors behind certain contagious diseases. It was not until later that I began to fit my early ecologic studies into the existing epidemiologic investigations.[6]

As an ecologic study, the focus was on the relationship of man to his natural and social environment. Park,[7] who may be regarded as the founder of human ecology, saw competition and communication as the two processes representing the core of man's existence. Competition was ever present, impersonal, and central in accounting for how man distributed himself in his physical environment. It was also the process that separated men from each other while communications was the process that brought them together. Thus, the competition present in the social order was not permitted to work itself out to its ultimate end, but rather was arrested by the social or moral order that emerged from the communicating process. Within the social order, the struggle was intense. Some men fought their way to positions of power and influence. Others assisted them, and still others had to be content with positions of powerlessness. Still others could be regarded as the failures; criminals, prostitutes, the insane, the poverty-stricken, the mentally retarded, in short those people who either rebelled from or could not be fitted into the social structure. This was the picture of man's lot provided by the theory of human ecology.

Within this context, the central criticism that the social scientist directed toward this study was statistical. It was argued that rates in certain communities, such as skid row and rooming house areas, were not valid because they were based on a population that turned over three and four times a year. However, even when the population in these areas was multiplied by three or four, the rates still remained high. Another criticism was that the decline in rates from the center to the periphery of the city might not be valid because the differences between contiguous communities were not statistically significant. However, this was corrected by joining such communities together to increase the population base, and so the gradient tendency that had been noted seemed to hold up.

While these psychiatric and sociologic criticisms had validity at the time, they lost much of their cogency in light of the tremendous social changes that have taken place over the past 50 years. Such changes have undermined the ecologic conceptions of community growth and decline.

The theory of human ecology that was the framework of our early studies might still be useful if human communities had continued to develop, grow, and decline without human plan or intervention. However, planning and intervention operated to change the original distribution patterns. It is such changes that have provided a new perspective for the interpretation of epidemiologic and ecologic studies of mental disorders. It is impossible to touch on all of the social forces that have been operating during these past years, and I will attempt only to pinpoint the most significant ones.

I suggest that a total conjoint force operating during the past half century to produce tremendous changes in our social organization is found in the linkage of science, technology, and federal power. This trilogy has been successful in introducing elements productive of vast changes into our community life. While I cannot cover all of these elements, I will discuss some that are crucial to our concern, namely, the interpretation of epidemiologic studies of mental disorder.

First, I am referring primarily to the development of computers, which have speeded, changed, and innovated human communication; to the development of the jet airplane, which has made every spot on the globe a matter of hours away; the perfection of television has made it possible to bring the great diversity of cultural settings into our living rooms; the entire social security program which has assured a minimum income for most persons in their later years; and to the federal support of various urban demolition and renewal programs that have changed the whole character and structure of selected neighborhoods and community life. Finally, I refer to the role of federal power in advancing the civil rights of all minorities: blacks, hispanics, Indians, and women.

I wish now to consider each one of these developments that have become part of our community life during the past half century and some of the resulting consequences. If one looks at the revolution in communication that computers, television, and jet airplanes have made possible, one is struck by the fact that much of that communication can take place with a minimum of personal contact. For example, the introduction of teaching machines in the schools, the widespread use of computers in business and government, the development of automatic factories, and the organization of various pressure groups overnight are only a few ways that these new technologies are changing our world and keeping human contact to a minimum.

The social security program has also produced changes that have weakened community life. Let me refer to two such developments. First, the minimum security benefits enable persons above 65 to live more independently from their families. What was once a family obligation to care for the elderly has now been passed on to the government. The social security program in conjunction with Medicare and the new policy of emptying the mental hospitals has stimulated the development of nursing homes—the new way of handling the elderly in our society. Further, the social security program has been a factor in reducing the populations of skid rows in our cities so that currently skid row is an "open asylum" and a collecting ground for those misfits, the psychological maladjusted, and physically handicapped who for one reason or another are ineligible for social security benefits.

A vast federal urban renewal program developed in the 1950s provided a mechanism for clearing selected urban slums, disrupting old stable neighborhoods, and scattering people to other areas in the cities where they knew no one and had minimum social contact.[8]

These programs have generally been supported by local city planning groups which, while they talk of people's needs, largely ignore them in practice.

Finally, the exercise of federal power in the civil rights area has often stimulated a new social consciousness in members of minority groups. This has been especially true with respect to our black citizens who have flooded our schools and colleges and have found jobs in many organizations which previously never hired them. This new consciousness is manifested also in the increased numbers of blacks and other minorities who have run for public office and who increasingly have been elected and re-elected. Through this new political power and through the flight of whites to the suburbs, they have often obtained political control in certain cities. This has been all to the good, but difficulties arise because while they have political power, they frequently lack the essential economic power that is also necessary to govern.

This new social consciousness among minority groups has been supported by federal power. How far and how fast can the federal government move in support of the value of nondiscrimination before it weakens certain elements of current social organization? In the rules and regulations developed to support this value, federal power has challenged the older principle that morality cannot be legislated. But in making the challenge, the government has demonstrated that such legislation has its educational use and has prevented certain acts of discrimination that would have happened if the legislation was not present. The problem really is how can we strike a balance between the achievement of equal rights for all citizens and the preservation of those institutional structures essential for the maintenance of order.

This new extention of civil liberties has also been felt with respect to the mentally ill as state after state, sometimes as a result of federal pressure, has attempted to empty the mental hospitals and to return the care and treatment of the mentally ill to the local communities. When one adds up the various developments in the area of civil liberties, one might argue that during the past half century the mechanism for social control has moved from coercion to a kind of psychological humanism wherein control is obtained through several types of therapy. This does not mean that force is neither operative nor used by the government, but rather that the attempt to secure accommodation is made through a more humanistic social engineering.[9]

These changes have brought about a partially planned social structure in contrast to the earlier unplanned structure. This shift provides a different background for viewing the distribution of mental diseases in the community in contrast to that provided by the laissez faire ecologic structure. Consequently, the current interpretation of rate patterns must consider a context of unstable neighborhoods, minimal communication, a partial economic security for most persons, and a constant pressure from various minority groups that demand their constitutional rights.

Thus, these changes that I have described undermine the confidence concerning the interpretation of the distribution of rate patterns that was much evidenced in the 1930s. For example, at the time the distribution pattern of schizophrenic rates was viewed as a product of social disorganization that engulfed the residents of communities at the center of the city. Other epidemiologic studies at the time also were interpreted as supporting the possibility of an environmental cause of mental disorder in opposition to the more popular genetic explanation.[10]

While no definitive statement could be made then about etiology, there was a tendency to point out that certain social milieus were conducive to the development of schizophrenia. While the crucial factor continued to elude us, at least the distribution pattern suggested where to look. One made the assumption that persons who became schizophrenic were born, grew up, and continued to live in the same community. While this assumption could hardly be granted even then, it was often overlooked in the attempt to give some meaning to the distribution patterns. At the time, the uneven and random distribution of the manic-depressive psychosis seemed to provide a unique support for viewing certain communities as productive of schizophrenics. Thus, Faris and I argued from a sociologic perspective that the isolation of the person might be a key process in the development of a schizophrenic disorder. While that was suggested as a hypothesis, it was elevated by certain sociologists as an established proposition about the social basis of this disorder. Studies began to appear, some supporting and others critical of our findings with respect to schizophrenia.

However, let me turn for a moment to some of the consequences that grew out of these social changes. They are important because they undermine the smugness of our earlier interpretation of schizophrenic rate patterns. One of the earlier criticisms emphasized that correlations using communities as units was one thing, while correlations using individuals as units was quite another matter. This was the ecologic fallacy and was a fair criticism of our earlier study. There we had attempted to make certain inferences about individual behavior and experiences on the basis of the correlations of the rate distribution with other community variables.[11] This was patently unsound and represented a word of caution to social scientists before jumping from community structures to individual human experiences. Specifically, the criticism suggested that a rate distribution indicated where to look rather than what to look for. What to look for had to be sought in other types of study designs.

A second consequence was to call attention to social mobility. Certain studies attempted to show either that excessive mobility was productive of mental derangement or that mental derangement tended to lead to excessive social mobility[12] Which was the case? On the ecologic level, social mobility was viewed as a collective factor in the attempt to show that excessive mobility indicated an area where the rate of maladjustment was bound to be high. The findings were inconclusive, and the general conclusion eventually was that mobility had little meaning with respect to mental illness.[13] This factor, however, began to appear in a new light when examined with respect to the distribution of schizophrenics and suggested that the mobility of a schizophrenic case was a result of certain selective factors both in the person and in the community that might account for his location in geographical space.[14]

A third consequence was a change in attitudes toward mental illness. The tendency to view the mentally ill with fear and horror and as products of supernatural influences began to give way in the popular mind to more tolerant, human, and naturalistic ways of looking at the development of mental illness. This meant a marked increase in community tolerance for the mentally ill.[15] Community tolerance, then, was a factor which prevented immediate commitment when a mental disturbance was detected and thus delayed entrance into official statistics.

This changing public attitude, the frustration of psychiatrists treating the psychoses, and the increase in civil liberties for the mentally ill have all helped to produce what I have called the "widening definition of mental illness." Patients who formerly would not even be considered mentally ill are now caught in the psychiatric net. Under the umbrella of mental disturbance, the psychiatrist is expected to treat and manage not only bona-fide psychotics, but also the psychologically maladjusted, various forms of deviant behavior, and those persons nurtured by unacceptable subcultures in our society. This widening definition means that any person who will not go along with or sets himself against institutional regulations might run the risk of being defined as mentally ill. It seems clear to me that faith in the democratic ethos should make it impossible to view verbal and legal challenges to sacred traditions or institutional authority as signs of mental illness.

Another consequence of the changes to which I have referred is the increase in the various kinds of agencies that deal with the mentally ill. This development, as I have pointed out elsewhere, has become a nightmare to any epidemiologist concerned with getting a complete count of all cases or a given type of case.

Thus, the clinical distinctions that have been thought with some assurance to exist, tend to become blurred, shifting, and uncertain, and the emphasis is placed on helping the person even though one does not know what his condition is or what is behind it.

This increase of agencies has been accompanied by a mad rise of new types of therapy. Whether or not the current drug culture is responsible for emphasizing heightened levels of consciousness, there is no doubt that many people have taken this message to heart and seek out various kinds of therapies, collective and otherwise, that will provide consciousness-raising experiences. Therapy becomes something which everybody should experience, and the atmosphere is created that enables a person without any shame or sensitivity to say that he needs therapeutic help. The implications of this shift are so far reaching it is difficult to enumerate them all. It is probably sufficient to say that the tremendous number of new therapies gives some idea of the thirst for new experiences and heightened awareness of reality. Rather than viewing them as a form of psychiatric help, it would seem more meaningful to view them as tentative groupings for the close and intimate relationships that are denied persons in the technologic and computerized society that has emerged.

The policy of decentralizing many of the older social control mechanisms has tended to produce more rigid bureaucratic forms. This means that while the old traditional mental hospital had a personal bureaucracy, the new community agencies have had to develop a more rigid bureaucracy, the new community agencies have had to develop a more rigid bureaucracy to show that they are capable of handling a new and unmfamiliar task. This, of course, means that the democratic and civil liberty values that were behind such decentralization and were thought to be supportive of an eclectic therapeutic program turn out to be of little help in the emerging, bureaucratic mental health structures.

Finally, these changes have stimulated a search for new interpretations of the rate patterns. The criticism directed against viewing them as supports for societal causation theories has resulted in investigators taking a second look and so finding more sociologically grounded interpretations than was originally the case. Thus, some investigators have viewed rate variations in terms of the number of beds available at different times and places.[16] Buck[17] sees them as a reflection of community tolerance; Hare and others [18] have emphasized a voluntary segregation. Clausen and Kohn[19] view differential rate variations as a reflection of city size; Dunham[20] sees rate variation patterns for schizophrenics as a result of a social selection process; and Rowitz and Levy[21] speak of rate variations in differences between communities in the use of mental hospitals.

It is our contention that these social changes and their consequences have tended to produce a vague and uncertain psychiatric terrain that makes it difficult both to conduct epidemiologic studies of mental illness and to interpret their findings. The epidemiologic study of mental illness or any other illness for that matter is very much dependent upon some clear conception of the entity being studied. When this entity is vague, uncertain, and defined differently at various times and places, such studies tend to become meaningless. The eagerness to help people, the extended ease with which mental ill health is indicated, and the democratic desire to insure the civil liberties of people defined as mentally ill make it almost impossible to conduct meaningful epidemiologic investigations. When such studies are conducted, however, they can still serve as the best instrument available for the assessment of mental health needs. The future of such studies and their value for need assessment will depend on the development of more carefully constructed diagnostic types. This will come about when the consequences of changes that we have considered have run their course and the social structure develops a new settled and orderly organization supportive of more rational decisions.

## NOTES

1.  Faris, R. E. L., & Dunham, H. W. *Mental disorders in urban areas.* Chicago: University of Chicago Press, 1939.

2.  Scheff, T. *Being mentally ill.* Chicago: Aldine Publishing Co., 1966. (See also: The moral career of the mental patient. *Psychiatry: Journal for the Study of Interpersonal Processes,* (May) 1959, 22.

3. Dohrenwend, B. & Dohrenwend, B. The problem of validity in field studies of psychological disorder. *Journal of Abnormal Psychology*, 1965, *70*, 52–59.

4. Dunham, H. W. *Community and schizophrenia*. Detroit: Wayne State University Press, 1965. Pp. 80–84.

5. Myerson, A. Review of mental disorders in urban areas. *American Journal of Psychiatry*, (January) 1941, *96*, 995–997.

6. Dunham, H. W. Psychiatric epidemiology in medical ecology. *Archives of General Psychiatry*, (January 1966, *14*, 1–19.

7. Park, R. Human ecology. *American Journal of Sociology*, (July) 1931, *37*, 1–15.

8. Gans, H. *The urban villagers*. New York: The Free Press, 1962.

9. Goode, W. J. The place of force in human society. *American Sociological Review*, (October) 1972, *37*, 507–519.

10. MacDermott, W. R. The topographical distribution of insanity. *British Medical Journal*, (September 26) 1908, *2*, 950.

11. Robinson, W. D. Ecological correlations and the behavior of individuals. *American Sociological Review*, (June) 1950, *15*, 351–357.

12. Tietze, C., Lemkau, P., & Cooper, M. Personal disorder and spatial mobility. *American Journal of Sociology*, (July) 1942, *48*, 129–139.

13. Murphy, H. B. M. Social change and mental health. In *Causes of mental disorder: A review of epidemiological knowledge*. New York: Milbank Memorial Fund, 1951. Pp. 280–329.

14. Dunham, H. W. *Community and schizophrenia*. op. cit. p. 230.

15. Buck, C., Wanklin, J. M., & Hobbs, G. F. Symptom analysis of rural-urban differences in first admission rates. *Journal of Nervous and Mental Diseases*, (July) 1955, *122*, 80–82.

16. Odegaard, O. The distribution of mental disease in Norway. *Acta Psychiatrica et Neurologica*, 1945, *20*, 247–284.

17. Buck, C., et al, *op. cit.* (See also: Analysis of regional differences in mental illness. *Journal of Nervous and Mental Diseases*, (July) 1955, *122*, 73–79).

18. Gerard, D., & Houston, L. G. Family setting and the social ecology of schizophrenia. *Psychiatric Quarterly*, (January) 1953, *27*, 90–101. (See also: Hare, E. H. Family setting and the urban distribution of schizophrenia. *Journal of Mental Science*, (October) 1956, 102).

19.  Clausen, J. A., & Kohn, M. L. The relation of schizophrenia to the social structure of a small city. In B. Pasamanick (Ed.), *Epidemiology of mental disorder.* American Association for the Advancement of Science, Publication No. 60 (1959), Washington, D. C.

20.  Dunham, H. W. *op. cit.*

21.  Levy, L., & Rowitz, L. *The ecology of mental disorder.* New York: Behavior Publications, 1973.

*Chapter 3*

# THE RELEVANCE OF EPIDEMIOLOGY
# TO NEED ASSESSMENT STRATEGIES

*Ben A. Locke*

When I first began preparing this chapter, I thought I knew nothing about need assessment. I now realize that if epidemiologists and need assessors are not kin, we are at least in the same ball park and usually playing on the same team.

Assumptions are in order. Personally I assume epidemiology as that which epidemiologists do. After wading through a plethora of definitions and descriptions, it seems to me that need assessment is what need assessors do.

Those of us engaged in either enterprise have many virtues in common. We are action oriented; we seek sensible solutions to today's problems; we attempt to provide quantifiable and scientific answers. Indeed, epidemiology is considered the scientific arm of public health.

While we may be kissing cousins, we also have our differences. Differences in philosophy and style determine how we define a problem and therefore impact upon the strategies for solution. At this point I had best present one of the more professional definitions of epidemiology.[1]

> In a current definition, epidemiology is the study of the
> distribution and determinants of states of health in human

populations. This definition has room for most present day activities of epidemiologists. Some prefer to add that these activities are for the purpose of the prevention, surveillance, and control of health disorders in population. This addition emphasizes a determinant of health and medicine, namely, such conscious intervention in health matters as societies elect to undertake.

Throughout this chapter, I hope to indicate areas conducive to collaboration and those where divergent needs or demands necessitate separate strategies.

What we share in common are surveys, if we use the term in a broad sense.[1]

In saying that elaboration of the "survey" method is the core of epidemiologic method, we affirm its common ground with the other disciplines involved in the study of society. States of health do not exist in a vacuum apart from people. People form societies, and any study of the attributes of people is also a study of the manifestations of the form, the structure, and the processes of social forces. On the other hand, epidemiology's segregation from other studies of society in its choice of states of health as dependent variable, gives it common ground with other medical sciences. It differs from other medical sciences in that the unit of study is populations and not individuals.

One use of surveys is descriptive, to set out norms and limits of the distribution of variables in numerical terms. Surveys quantify the attributes of populations, of environments, and of periods of time. They provide an understanding of a selected problem, its size, its nature, among whom and where it is to be found, and, indeed, whether the problem exists. In epidemiology, there are the distributions of states of health referred to in our original definition of epidemiology. A second use of surveys is explanatory or analytical—to compare different populations in relation to environments and trends in time and to account for the variations between them. In epidemiology this is the study of the determinants referred to in our definition.

Despite much useful work by several disciplines in survey research, many methodologic problems remain. Indeed, rising costs and falling response rates serve to exacerbate existing problems. When can we use mail or phone interviews rather than the costly face-to-face technique? Perhaps out of desperation, there are some who now allege that sensitive data can best be collected by phone, that the respondent feels freer when not physically facing the interviewer and seeing the responses recorded.

But what is a sensitive question? About 40 years ago I volunteered to collect data for a study about driving habits and accidents. Although common now, it was uncommon then to have detailed questions about one's sexual activities and attitudes. My first respondent was a woman, and I was certain as I began that section that I would be thrown out of her home. I was wrong. I heaved a sigh of relief and about one or two minutes later came to the last question. I could not believe my ears when I heard "Aren't you being intimate? That is between the IRS and me and no concern of yours." Yes, the last question (wisely) was about income which, as you know, is still a sensitive question.

Perhaps one major difference between an epidemiologic and a need assessment approach is the degree to which one feels comfortable in accepting an individual's appraisal of his or her health. As an epidemiologist who participated in the control of tuberculosis by means of mass x-ray surveys, I am acutely aware of how many people felt well yet had TB—that is, sputum positive active TB.

A few years ago, the Center for Epidemiologic Studies of the National Institutes for Mental Health (NIMH) supported two community household surveys. We were interested in determining how many individuals evidenced "depression."[2-4] Of those that scored high in depressive symptomatology, about one-third denied being depressed.

Similarly, we should have reservations about asking patients' satisfaction with services as a means of assessing medical care. Often, patients' responses are based on reasons irrelevant to the issue, and consequently conclusions may place its users in an erroneous zone.

Again, allow me to be anecdotal. When I was the Director of Research and Evaluation for a university's Community Mental

Health Center, we assigned a psychiatrist to the Medical School's Community Health Program. Briefly, care to the local population was provided by rotating residents on a quarterly basis, and patients were very satisfied. An individual with stomach problems was promptly and enthusiastically taken care of, and four or five months later the back problem was equally well handled, and then the arm and then the foot and so forth. When I left, that psychiatrist was writing a paper, the gist of which was that the fat folders (medical records) represented misdiagnosed patients, who were truly psychiatric patients being treated for their presenting somatic complaints. Yet those patients were happy with their health services.

There is also evidence that patients may be satisfied with physicians who have been treating them for their condition for 5, 10, or more years, and I do not mean for such long-term illnesses as diabetes. In short, patient and physician can establish a comfortable relationship that may not result in the best medical care. Epidemiologists and need assessors should not shun the patient, but they have to consider criteria other than or in addition to the patient in evaluating service needs and efficacy.

Dr. Murrell[5] writes:

> (t)he basic output of a needs assessment is information. The purpose for which this information is used typically concerns program evaluation, program planning, or program development. Needs assessment information, therefore, should be relevant to program decisions and to program managers.

Thus,

> (n)eeds assessment can play an important part in decisions affecting the distribution of a community mental health center's resources. The process of assessing needs can reveal zones of potentially high need for service within a catchment area, and can uncover segments of the populations inadvertently overlooked in the course of providing services. A reliable needs assessment study may thus provide a mandate for change in a center's staff, service emphasis, budget, or location of satellite services.[6]

Here is where differences in philosophy may result in differing emphases. It has been stated that[7]

(i)n the field of mental health, epidemiology can serve the following purposes:

(1)  to assess the prevalence of different types of mental ill-health in a population as a basis for the prevention, treatment and control of diseases;

(2)  to uncover associations between population characteristics and disease that may clarify the origins of mental disorder;

(3)  to test etiologic hypotheses originating from laboratory or clinical studies;

(4)  to assess rates of spontaneous recovery in order to evaluate the effectiveness of preventive measures.

Let me elaborate on that from another World Health Organization report:[8]

The epidemiological approach in psychiatry can be used for two main purposes, which are, of course, to a certain extent interrelated. It can be employed in what may be called "operational research" to elicit facts about treated and untreated disease in the community which are needed for the intelligent administration of psychiatric services. It can also be used in clinical work to discover those features of the habits, organization or environments of human populations which may affect the onset or course of mental disorders, and to assess their relative importance in the etiological structure of such conditions.

Public health administrators must have estimates of both present and future demands and needs for psychiatric services, and these requirements differ according to geographical conditions, the social organization, and the age and structure of particular populations. Moreover, they must study the functional efficiency of psychiatric services, existing or planned in relation to these demands and needs. The epidemiological approach will therefore be necessary for assessing the prevalence and incidence of psychiatric disorders in specified population groups, the use made of existing services by the population concerned, and the changes in this use that are likely to result from projected changes in the existing arrangements. This type of approach is clearly of special importance in those areas where psychiatric services are not yet either numerous or varied. But it is hardly less important in other regions where the services are already more or less highly developed, since the progress of psychiatry demands constant adaptive changes—affecting both material facilities and staffing—in the organization of services.

The role of epidemiology in clinical research is to seek clues to the causation of disease. The comparison of the disease experience of population groups in relation to various factors—time, space, age, occupation, social situation, etc.—should allow the contrasting of groups which are particularly affected and to suggest etiological factors which might explain specific susceptibility to diseases, or the forms in which they are manifested. When such factors can be changed by human action, methods of disease control based on their probable role can be put to the test by trials in the field. This sort of approach is clearly of less immediate utility than operational research. In the long run, however, its practical importance may be even greater. In fact, only when the "natural history" of a disease—that is, its evolution over long periods in clearly defined circumstances—has been determined in a particular population will there be possibilities for devising measures for its control and prevention which are not based on mere speculation.

It would thus seem that need assessment serves primarily to deploy agency resources to maximize services in terms of patients receiving such benefits. To the epidemiologist, prevention and/or control of disease is primary. In public health, a patient represents failure.

My hope is to present a convincing argument that prevention is practical and can be combined with many present programs and activities. But first let me review the current advantages, as I see them, in appraising community services which need assessors have over epidemiologists.

The epidemiologist engaged in etiologic research and seeking causative or associative factors must worry about response rate. Lately, response rates have been dropping; we seem to be settling for 70 percent or less, yet obviously the missing 30 percent poses serious problems in determining association. For needs assessment purposes, this may pose as serious a problem. The 30 percent may well be a group that will not use your services as currently provided.

While both epidemiologists and need assessors conduct community surveys on random samples of the population to determine incidence and prevalence, the degree of detail and extensiveness of independent variables needed by need assessors is substantially less than that needed by epidemiologists. Therefore, the number of respondents, as well as total interviewing time, can be less.

Prevalence is defined in the following ways:

> ... as the number of cases of disease present in a population at a given time; incidence is the number of new cases occurring within a specified period.[7]
> Prevalence depends on the rates of inception of a disease, recovery, and recurrence, and on the mortality among its victims.[9]
> Incidence, on the other hand, measures the rate at which new cases are added to the total of sick persons, and is dependent on the balance between resistance of the population and those stresses—biological, cultural and psychological—that evoke mental disorder.[10]

The importance of these relationships was emphasized by Kramer who developed models that[9]

> ... demonstrated a fact well known to persons trained in epidemiology, but not to many of the newcomers to the field of psychiatric epidemiology—that equal prevalence rates for a given mental disorder in two population groups does not necessarily mean equal incidence or equal duration. Since

prevalence is a function of incidence and duration, differences—or for that matter, a lack of differences—in prevalence rates can be accounted for by differences either in incidence, duration, or in both.

However, the immediate problem is having an adequate and acceptable means of measuring mental disorders in the community. We are all aware of past efforts and current criticisms and problems in attempting to use measures from the past. The problem is well stated by Kramer:[9]

It is high time for the various researchers who have carried out community surveys, developed psychiatric screening techniques, and developed procedures for improving the comparability of psychiatric diagnosis to be brought together to determine whether their research has improved the prospects for developing standardized casefinding techniques for use in community surveys of the prevalence of psychiatric disorder. If prospects are promising, then recommendations should be made as to next steps in our attempts to solve this problem. If they are not promising, then this should be stated clearly. The same experts could also review the situation with respect to the possibilities of developing uniform procedures for determining incidence and make a similar evaluation. Such an assessment of the status of case finding for mental disorders would be helpful in putting into perspective the possibilities of our collecting systematic morbidity data on the mental disorders other than those based on the records of patients admitted to psychiatric facilities.

Recognizing that as a problem, the Division of Biometry and Epidemiology did just that: We convened the proponents of the four major new systems for use in making differential diagnoses. Rather than using a global assessment scale, the newer instruments attempted, to provide specific diagnoses.

Our need to make that determination resulted from approval for the Center for Epidemiologic Studies to initiate a major program entitled the Epidemiologic Catchment Area (ECA)

Program. One major part of this program is conducting community (household) surveys as well as surveys in settings such as prisons, nursing homes, and homes for the aged.

But even if we solved the measurement issue, thorny problems remain. One major problem involves knowing which of our designated cases would see themselves as cases and would also agree that they need and will use mental health services.

In a study that we conducted in two communities to measure depressive symptomatology, we found nearly 20 percent above our cutoff score.[2] Only 11 percent, however, responded "yes" to the question about feeling that they had an emotional problem. Of these, only 7 percent indicated that they wanted help, yet only half actually obtained it.[11] Although the exact figures vary, other studies have shown similar results, namely, only a small segment of those deemed in need of psychiatric services were actually willing to use them.

For example, in "Americans View Their Mental Health" the investigators found that 60 percent of those who felt they had emotional problems and needed help actually obtained it.[12] In a study in New York City, 47 percent had emotional problems, but only 9 percent obtained help.[13] One study that reported that 30 percent obtained help involved a prepaid medical care plan in which only 10 percent admitted having emotional problems.[14]

Given these findings, one must wonder about the myth that mental illness coverage in any proposed National Health Insurance program would break the bank. For example, a study of the auto workers—the first large wage-earning group in this country to be insured for mental health care—showed[15]

> . . . a definite tendency among the workers to avoid professional mental health care. Almost 27 percent of the workers said they would either do nothing, ignore the problems, or cope with the problems themselves.

Only "about 14 percent said they would seek help from a mental health profession."[15]

In this report, it was speculated that stigma attached to mental illness is influential in the low use of the mental health service system. This speculation is substantiated by the work of the President's Commission on Mental Health. In reporting on that Commission's findings, then First Lady Rosalynn Carter stated:[16]

> ... one thing that was pervasive in every hearing and every discussion we had was the stigma of mental illness. It is so important. People in our country still attach a stigma to mental illness, and I think we are going to have to overcome that before we can see real progress in the treatment of the mentally afflicted.

Both epidemiologists and need assessors must be concerned about the issue of stigma not only in how it affects service planning but also in the possible biasing of responses when we seek basic information. And, obviously, we must seek a better understanding of the phenomenon so we can remove the cause.

Without minimizing the need to solve problems inherent in community surveys, valuable need assessment data can be obtained from physicians' offices and other medical settings for a reasonable investment. Although estimates vary, in most places over half the adult population are seen by a physician during the year, usually more than once, and many are well known by their physicians. In a study Gardner and I conducted in Monroe County, New York, 17 percent of 11,144 white patients aged 15 years old or older were perceived by their physicians to have psychiatric problems.[17] In another study in Monroe County, New York, involving general hospital clinics, physicians reported 22 percent of 1,413 patients aged 15 years and older to have emotional disorders.[18] Remember, these are diagnoses made by physicians who are not psychiatrists. It is my contention that in such settings some of the simpler scales, either self-administered symptom checklists like the SCL-90 or the CES-D or otherwise administered such as the GHO, would pick up many missed cases of "mental disorders" to the benefit of both patient and physician.

While such endeavors lack the elegance of community surveys and do not permit easy generalizations as to prevalence and incidence, they do furnish useful information for program planning of services as well as for consultation and education.

Let me quickly run through several other epidemiologic strategies that could be relevant in need assessment work. When asked why he robbed banks, Willie Sutton allegedly responded "because that's where the money is." Well, epidemiologists have found that given a case (a patient), it is worthwhile to examine the entire family. Although this procedure is based on the contagious disease model, it seems desirable to try it out experimentally to evaluate its usefulness.

This technique is one of several aimed at addressing the high-risk group. Based on utilization data and other relevant data, certain categories of the citizenry can be classified as high risk, meaning they would furnish a high yield of cases or potential patients. Examples of such specific populations are the unemployed, the bereaved, postpartum women, and women undergoing unwanted pregnancies.

We are exploring research strategies that will furnish us with information that will enable us to promote programs of prevention among the separated and divorced. Such planned intervention we call experimental epidemiology inasmuch as we cannot claim that the outcome will be successful. But even failure furnishes knowledge that aids in moving the field forward.

I will not discuss the area of census data and demographic profiles in detail here. But I will make a plea for obtaining occupational data as part of the routine intake or devising a plan that would allow you to access such data from the Social Security System. Without endorsing the analytic approach, I call to your attention a study entitled "Occupational Incidence Rates of Mental Health Disorders."[19] In a study that I did in collaboration with Mancuso, we found carbon disulphide to be implicated as a cause of suicide among a group of workers.[20] Actually, our hypothesis was that $CS_2$ caused depression. Not having access to depression data, we used suicide data that made the hypothesis more difficult to substantiate.

Let me reiterate that prevention—primary, secondary, and tertiary—underlies all efforts of epidemiologists. Tertiary prevention is aimed at reducing the degree of impairment and chronicity caused by disease. Secondary prevention has as its objective the *restoration* of full functioning as soon as possible, and we assume that early case-finding aids and abets such efforts.

Primary prevention is the holy grail of epidemiologists and should be for need assessors. To the epidemiologist, prevalence statistics, while useful, must provide additional data about factors contributing to becoming a case so that programs of intervention and prevention can be developed. As Dr. Turns so succinctly put it as the First Conference on Need Assessment in Health and Human Services, "The raison d'etre of epidemiology and public health, after all, is to prevent illness, not to measure it over and over again."[21]

In answer to the question "where will the resources come from?" Dr. Brown, former Director of the National Institute of Mental Health, said,[22]

> If there are to be no new resources to meet this objective, then either it cannot be operationalized despite the development of scientific knowledge, or the resources for direct treatment services will be impinged upon. This latter suggestion implies a sense of competition that inevitably turns out to be highly dysfunctional. Public health theory suggests that prevention is not only a sounder approach to health maintenance than treatment, but also, in the long run, less expensive.

My response to those of you who wonder who will pay for prevention is that the public is now paying dearly for treatment and that an ounce of prevention is worth a pound of cure. But I will be more realistic.

Several times I have heard Dr. Bryant, Chairman of the President's Commission on Mental Health, speak about the preliminary and final reports. What he said is consonant with Mrs. Carter's response in a radio interview to a question on prevention. I quote:[16]

> Well, as a matter of fact, when I gave Jimmy the report, we didn't have a recommendation about prevention, and that was the first thing he asked me . . . So that will be in the April 1 report. It is very important and we are studying it carefully.

Indeed, given the expressed interest of Mr. Califano, the Secretary of Health, Education and Welfare, with regard to efforts to reduce smoking, it is most likely that mental health professionals will need to become more involved in trying to understand why people, particularly young people, resort to or participate in antisocial or self-destructive behavior.

The following excerpt expresses this concept well.[23]

> The social epidemiologist is uniquely equipped to inquire into behavior changes which could affect reduction in disease. This is because he is aware of social situations which can produce disease and knows how to study ways of effecting behavior change. Several traditions of the behavioral sciences can suggest hypotheses to the social epidemiologist interested in conducting what we might call preventive research. Anthropologists have studied in the area of diffusion of innovations in primarily preliterate societies. Rural sociologists have investigated approaches to studying acceptance and rejection of agricultural innovation, such as high yield seed, fertilizers, and the like. Psychologists have studied behavior change, primarily in small groups and in individuals, and sociologists, too, have carried out research on behavior change and the diffusion of innovations. Thus, there is a growing body of literature as to variables related to behavior change. This could suggest studies of ways to effect behavior which would put the findings of epidemiology to work to reduce the incidence of disease. It may ultimately be possible to understand ways of persuading individuals not to smoke cigarettes, to use seat belts, to obtain cervical cytology, to reduce their weight, and the like. This is such a logical thing for social epidemiogists to undertake, they are located so strategically in the social situation to do it, and they are so well equipped to do it, or can get the needed knowledge, that they will increasingly extend their inquiries from social factors in the prevention of disease. I hope this interest comes sooner rather than later.

And I hope all need assessors join us in this grand effort.

## Notes

1.   Susser, M. *Causal thinking in the health sciences: Concepts and strategies of epidemiology.* New York: Oxford University Press, 1973.

2.  Comstock, G. W., & Helsing, K. J. Symptoms of depression in two communities. *Psychological Medicine,* 1976, *6,* 551–563.

3.  Radloff, L. S. The CES-D Scale: A self-report depression scale for research in the general population. *Applied Psychological Medicine,* 1977, *1*(3), 385–401.

4.  Weissman, M. M., et al. Assessing depressive symptoms in five psychiatric populations: A validation study. *American Journal of Epidemiology,* 1977, *106*(3), 203–214.

5.  Murrell, S. A. Utilization of needs assessment for community decision-making. *American Journal of Community Psychology,* 1977, *5*,(4), 461–468.

6.  Schwab, J. J., Warheit, G. J., & Fennell, E. Needs assessment methods for the community mental health center, *Evaluation,* 1975, *2*(2), 64.

7.  Lin, T., & Standley C. C. *The scope of epidemiology in psychiatry.* WHO Public Health Paper No. 16. Geneva: World Health Organization, 1962.

8.  World Health Organization *Epidemiology of mental disorders.* Technical Report Series No. 185. Geneva: World Health Organization, 1960.

9.  Kramer, M. Some perspectives on the role of biostatistics and epidemiology in the prevention and control of mental disorders. *The Milbank Memorial Fund Quarterly,* 1975, *53*(3), 297–336.

10. World Health Organization *Epidemiology of mental disorders.* Technical Report Series No. 185. Geneva: World Health Organization. 1960.

11. Cohen, J. B., Barbano, H., & Locke, B. Z. How biased is the tip of the iceberg? Characteristics of persons who seek help as a subset of persons who indicate they feel they are in need of help. *American Journal of Epidemiology,* 1976, *104*(3), 323–324.

12. Gurin, G., Veroff, J., & Feld, S. *Americans view their mental health: A nationwide interview survey.* New York: Basic Books, 1960.

13. Elinson, J. L., Padilla, E., & Perkins, M. E. *Public image of mental health services.* New York: Mental Health Materials Center, 1967.

14. Fink, R., Shapiro, S., & Goldensohn, S. S. Family physician referrals for psychiatric consultation and patient initiative in seeking care. *Social Science and Medicine,* 1970, *4,* 273–291.

15. Glasser, M. A., Duggan, T. J., & Hoffman, W. S. *Obstacles in the pathways to prepaid mental health care.* DHEW Publication No. (ADM) 76–383. Washington, D.C.: U.S. Government Printing Office, 1977.

16. Mental Health Matters. *An interview with Rosalynn Carter.* DHEW Publication No. (ADM) 78–582. Washington, D.C.: U.S. Government Printing Office, 1977.

17. Locke, B. A., & Gardner, E. A. Psychiatric disorders among the patients of general practitioners and internists. *Public Health Reports,* 1969, *84*(2), 167–173.

18. Rosen, B. M., et al. Identification of emotional disturbance in patients seen in general and medical clinics. *Hospital and Community Psychiatry,* 1972, *23*(12), 364–370.

19. Colligan, M. J., Smith, M. J., & Hurrell, J. J. Jr. Occupational incidence rates of mental health disorders. *Journal of Human Stress,* 1977, *3*(3), 34–39.

20. Mancuso, T. F., & Locke, B. Z. Carbon disulphide as a cause of suicide. *Journal of Occupational Medicine,* 1972, *14*(8), 595–606.

21. Turns, D. The measurement of health status. In R. A. Bell, M. Sundel, J. F. Aponte, & S. A. Murrell (Eds.), *Need Assessment in Health and Human Service,* Proceedings of the Louisville National Conference, 1976, pp. 80–90.

22. Brown, B. S. Critical issues for community mental health. *Journal of Social Welfare,* 1976, *3*(1), 7–21.

23. Graham, S. The sociological approach to epidemiology. *American Journal of Public Health,* 1974, *64*(11), 1046–1049.

Part II

# CONCEPTUAL AND THEORETICAL
# ISSUES IN NEED ASSESSMENT

## INTRODUCTION

This section covers topics, including issues and problems, related to the definition, identification, and determinants of need. Broskowski presents the basic concepts of general systems theory and applies them to the process of need assessment. He discusses the concept of environmental monitoring in examining the behavior of service provider organizations as open systems. Broskowski also draws systems implications for assessment of organizations and communities in relation to the prevention of illness and social disorders.

Nguyen, Attkisson, and Bottino examine basic assumptions underlying need identification and the issues and problems in the conceptualization of need. They propose a definition of unmet need, discuss its implications, and present a convergent analysis approach to need assessment. The authors also discuss differences and interrelationships between need assessment and program evaluation.

Turns and Newby examine factors related to the measurement of health status, including difficulties in arriving at adequate definitions of health and disease. They discuss major constraints on the development and usefulness of health status indicators, such as problems of validity and reliability. Turns and Newby caution need assessors against yielding to current pressures to provide health measurements for planning and service delivery without careful examination of the assumptions on which policies are based.

Dohrenwend presents a rationale for identifying social stressors related to serious health problems, focusing on stressful life events such as death in the family, divorce, job loss, or change of residence. She examines issues related to measuring the magnitude of stressful life events, as well as factors concerning the relation of risk of illness to the nature and magnitude of life events. Dohrenwend also discusses her study of contextual factors of anticipation and control on the occurrence of life events.

As indicated in the introduction to this volume, the field of need assessment can benefit from more clearly defined and operationalized concepts, particularly those addressing multiple, interrelated levels of needs. The editors feel that the authors in this section have made significant contributions in the conceptual and theoretical areas of need assessment.

*Chapter 4*

# THE APPLICATION OF GENERAL SYSTEMS THEORY IN THE ASSESSMENT OF COMMUNITY NEEDS

## *Anthony Broskowski*

As I have shifted my interests from the narrow category of mental health to the wider perspective of all human service programs, I have come to use general systems theory to conceptualize and guide my professional endeavors.[1-3] While theories of individual, group, and organizational behavior are still appropriate for specific problems, general systems theory has proven to be both stimulating and integrative for the tasks of planning, managing, and evaluating community-wide service delivery systems. It is this theoretical orientation, therefore, that I have brought to bear on the analysis of the need assessment process.

### GENERAL SYSTEMS THEORY

General systems theory proceeds on the assumption that there are principles isomorphic across all levels and types of systems, both living and nonliving. This chapter will focus on those concepts and principles of general systems that may help us to understand more fully the process of need assessment, including its planning, implementation, and the utilization of its findings.

General systems theorists address multiple levels of systems ranging from single cells through societies and international systems. For our purposes, we will restrict our analysis to the levels of individuals, families, organizations, and communities. Most frequently I will be referring to "the system" at the level of the single human service organization or network of organizations responsible for the actual planning and implementation of a need assessment. Later, however, I will speak about individuals and communities as systems for purposes of considering how need assessment efforts might be optimally focused for primary prevention and services integration.

### Some Basic Concepts of General Systems Theory

Before we can begin to relate general systems theory to the specific issues of need assessment, we must first review a number of basic concepts. This review, however, will be limited to those concepts of general systems theory which I see as most applicable to need assessment.*

*Systems defined.*    There are many definitions of system. We will use that of James Miller:[5]

*For a more thorough exposition of general systems theory and its uses, the reader should see Miller.[4,5] For examples of systems theory applied to organizational processes, the reader should see Baker,[6] Baker, Broskowski & Brandwein,[7] and Katz and Kahn.[8]

> A system is a set of interacting units with relationships among them. The word "set" implies that the units have some common properties, which is essential if they are to interact or have relationships. The state of each unit is constrained by, conditioned by, or dependent on the state of other units.

These units, generally referred to as subsystems, are linked as well as separated in various ways. Every system has a boundary that is more or less open to the environment. Every system must import matter and energy across its boundary to maintain itself as an organized structure and to carry out its productive processes. In the process of importing matter and energy, a system must usually convert them into some alternative form. For example, mechanical energy may be converted into electrical energy, which is further converted into light or heat waves.

By the first law of thermodynamics, energy is conserved, or never lost, in this process of conversion. Furthermore, energy and matter are equivalent, each being convertible to the other through the equation $E = mc^2$ ($c$ being the speed of light). Because of this equivalence, we will henceforth refer to them as matter-energy.

While the first law of thermodynamics addresses the issue of energy conservation, the second law emphasizes the direction of energy conversion and its general irreversibility. In the conversion of matter into energy, or vice versa, energy and matter move between relative states of order and disorder. But the direction of movement is not generally reciprocal or reversible. The second law states that matter, or organized systems, tends to move toward disorder, or entropy. Entropy increases over time as a system uses up its own available free energy. Therefore, without inputs of new matter and energy a system will move toward disorganization and decay.

Information is a special category of energy. It is patterned energy and is used by a system to organize the structural relationships among its own subsystems and to control the relative distribution of incoming matter-energy. It is generally of very low magnitude compared to the magnitude of matter-energy flow used for a system's productive work or maintenance. As the amount of incoming information increases, the rate of systemic entropy decreases. Wiener has shown that the formula used to measure information is equivalent to that which measures the negative condition of entropy, called negentropy.[9] A system, therefore, can reduce its rate of disorder and decay by importing sufficient amounts of new matter-energy and the information it needs to keep this matter-energy well organized.

Systems must do more than simply process an adequate quantity of information. The quality of information is critical. Ashby has formulated the Law of Requisite Variety, stating that a system must incorporate information of greater complexity than it actually needs for its own output or production.[10] That is, a system's informational input must be more complex than its output to maintain a steady state of negentropy. The surplus complexity is used (1) to restore internal breakdown or wear and (2) to support the development of new adaptive responses by providing a pool of surplus energy and information.

Matter, raw productive energy, and informational energy always flow together, although proportions vary depending on the process. The transmission of matter-energy can always convey some information, and the transmission of information will always require matter-energy. We will distinguish matter-energy from the special case of informational matter-energy or information. Any movement or change in matter-energy will be called *action*. Any movement or change in information will be called *communication*.

By highlighting the concepts of boundary permeability, matter-energy, and information flow, general systems theory focuses our attention on the importance of a system's environment. The environment exerts pressure on a system's boundary, and it is the source of the matter-energy and information needed for maintenance, productivity, and growth.

## ENVIRONMENTAL ADAPTATION AND MONITORING

Another general principle is that an adaptive system must differentiate its own internal subsystems and processes based, to some extent, on the characteristics of its environment. The system's environment can be conceptualized as differentiated, with different sectors having relatively different impact on or importance for different subsystems. These environmental sectors may vary in their complexity, their rate of change, and the certainty with which the system can determine environmental pressures or demands. The system must accommodate itself to these environmental differences by creating different specialized subsystems within itself. To remain current in its adaptation, the system must be able to detect environmental changes, especially if its environment is turbulent.

In brief, system survival, adaptation, productivity, efficiency, and effectiveness are dependent in part upon the abilities of the system to monitor its changing environment. In other words, "environmental monitoring" is the systemic process that we can liken to "need assessment" when we examine service provider organizations as open systems. Similarly, a management information system is analogous to the internal monitoring that a system must conduct to remain sensitive to its internal conditions. Finally, the program evaluation process is analogous to the systemic process of feedback: the monitoring of information about the effects of the system's outputs on its environment.

Before we examine environmental monitoring or need assessment more specifically, I would like to provide a few examples. While preparing this paper, I was struck by the numerous everyday examples of how large and small systems find it necessary to monitor their own environments. While only analogies, these examples may help to illustrate the general pervasiveness of the monitoring process.

The first example occurred to me while I sat in a cocktail lounge in Newport, Rhode Island, overlooking Narragansett Bay as a heavy fog suddenly rolled in. The boats coming into their moorings and docks were moving very cautiously, using lights, horns, and bells to signal their positions. The captains were most intent on scanning their environments. I was sure that many were sorry they had not had an earlier warning so they could have returned to port before it became so troublesome. Later I will return to this example as it illustrates specific phenomena of the monitoring process.

My teenage daughter engages in a ritual preparation of her school clothes. Her environmental monitoring includes not only weather forecasts but a few well placed phone calls to find out what her friends are wearing. This example illustrates nicely the importance of combining at least two different sources of information to perform a convergent analysis.

These examples illustrate environmental monitoring, but one might feel that they are a bit removed from need assessment. Need assessment sounds good, as though we are out looking for human needs to satisfy or for other people's problems to solve. Environmental monitoring, on the other hand, sounds self-serving, protective, and intended to help our own system to adapt or to avoid embarrassment or disaster. But that is precisely the motivation I detect in many cases where a need assessment is undertaken. I do not think it is an inappropriate motive, but I feel strongly that we ought to recognize it for what it is. Later I will return to this point in discussing some of the differences between two cases: (1) when a need assessment is done by an organization, as a system, on its own behalf, and (2) when a community, as a system, tries to assess its own internal conditions. While both cases may involve similar technologies, the motivations and uses of the information may differ greatly.

Upon receipt of information about its shifting environment, a system has four major options: do nothing, modify its internal structure or processes, modify its environment, or modify both. Systems tend toward stability and to resist change. Furthermore, they must be economical and efficient in their monitoring process. They therefore tend to monitor only those environmental sectors or variables that are most likely to require system adaptation or that are most amenable to modification by the system. For example, the sailboat captain will not bother to routinely monitor water temperature or salinity. These are technically feasible and easy measurements, but they make little difference for pleasure boating. Some commercial fishing boats, however, will monitor such characteritics. At the same time, both types of vessel will monitor general weather conditions and may use expensive radio equipment to extend their monitoring capacity beyond the limits of their immediate environments.

Early warning systems are environmental monitoring systems. Interestingly enough, differences between northern and southern rural communities in the use of early warning systems for tornadoes account for the major differences in their tornado death and injury rates. Differences in the use of inexpensive radio broadcast warnings and in the communities' response patterns after tornadoes struck were, in turn, traced to different beliefs as to whether or not tornadoes were inevitable, divine interventions, or natural phenomena to be mastered. Similarly, we can expect service agencies to vary the content and scope of their need assessment processes as a function of their perceived purpose and potential effectiveness. Most agencies will limit their assessment efforts along narrowly defined parameters related to their specialized services.

Here we face another intriguing dilemma. By the Law of Requisite Variety,[10] a system must process information of greater complexity than is needed for its productive purposes. Stated simply, the system must seek and incorporate diversity. But in the short run, many systems tend to drive out diversity because homogeneity can be more efficiently managed. In the long run, however, such homogenization and specialization can prove maladaptive. The point here is that agencies should remain open to assessments of needs that extend beyond their specialized service interests.

Since we have equated need assessment with environmental monitoring, let us focus our attention on some of the subsystems that process information:

1.  Information enters a system through the *boundary* which holds the other subsystems together, protects the system from environmental threats or stresses, and allows or excludes the entry of matter-energy and information. Boundaries can vary in flexibility, elasticity, and permeability.

2.  The *input transducer* is the sensory subsystem. It monitors the environment and brings information through the boundary, converting the energy form but not the content of that information for internal transmission. In this energy transduction, a certain degree of signal distortion or loss may result. Input transduction is illustrated by the intake worker who converts a client's words onto a piece of paper. Information is distorted if the words are changed and lost when voice inflections and gestures are not recorded.

3.  The *internal transducer* receives information from all other internal subsystems. Once again, the energy form of the signal may need to be converted before it can be passed on to other subsystems. If we equate the input transducer with the organizational process of need assessment, we would equate the internal transducer with the management information system (MIS). While the MIS is used to monitor internal activities, need assessment is used to monitor the organization's environment.[11]

4. The *channel and net* are the pathways or routes over which the information passes among subsystems.

5. The *decoder* receives information from the input or internal transducers and changes it into a common but private internal code. While the transducers change the information's energy form, the decoder changes its pattern or code. This process is illustrated by the coding of the written words of a patient on the intake worker's sheet into a restricted number of diagnostic codes. Further internal transduction may then take place if these codes are converted to keypunch cards or electrical signals on a computer tape.

6. The *associator* forms connections between items of information. These connections are not random or temporary but rather purposeful and enduring. This process may be carried out in an organization by its human members, or in some cases by equipment such as computers.

7. The *memory* stores information patterns or codes for varying amounts of time. Memory may be accomplished by such items as paper, computer tapes, and microfile or by the human memories of organizational members. Memories, of course, have varying capacity, accessibility, and rates of decay.

8. The *decider* is used for system control and integration. It receives information from all other subsystems, including internal and environmental sources, and transmits information codes to other subsystems, including those that process matter-energy. It thus controls the entire system. This subsystem is easily recognized as the executive or boss.

9. The *encoder* alters the information within the system from its private code to one that can be understood or interpreted by other systems in the environment. For example, public relations or advertising personnel frequently serve such functions.

10. The *output transducer* produces information outputs with an energy form that can be transmitted into the environment and received by other systems. Bro-

chures, newsletters, product manuals, films, and au-
diovisual tapes are examples of physical output transducers used by organizations. Theoretically, these outputs are used to stimulate or influence other systems in
the environment. For service systems with little in the
way of such matter-energy products as cars or washing
machines, information processing and production is
the major service or output for its clients.

It is not necessary to assume that these theoretical subsystems
exist as real and independent units or divisions within an organization. A single individual in an agency may carry out several
processes so quickly and smoothly that it is difficult to distinguish
them as separate subsystems. For the purposes of improving our
methods and uses of needs assessment, however, such distinctions are useful. (See Table 4-1).

From this analysis, one implication is obvious. From information collection to output, there are numerous opportunities
for changes in the amount and content of the original signal.
Parts of the signal will be lost in transduction and transmission.
Signal distortion may occur through filtration, suppression, or
amplification. Decoding and encoding may introduce additional
changes. Irrelevant noise or redundancy may be added. Some
signals can get mixed inappropriately with others. Some may be
stored in memory or stored so as to be irretrievable. It is a wonder
that systems can maintain any degree of signal fidelity.

Absolute signal fidelity, however, is seldom essential. Generally, the system must have environmental information that is at
least adequate in its fidelity, frequency, and complexity for immediate survival. Growth and long-term viability, however, will
add new demands. Important decisions require better information. As the environmental rate of change, complexity, or uncertainty increases, environmental monitoring efforts must also increase.

The process of need assessment must address identical
issues. How frequently, how accurately, and how extensively
must the need assessor monitor? It takes energy—in other words,
money—to monitor the environment. Energy devoted to monitoring is energy raken away from production. If systems do not

**Table 4-1    Critical Subsystems of Open Systems[4]**

| Matter-Energy Processing Subsystems | Subsystems which Process Both Matter-Energy and Information | Information- Processing Subsystems |
|---|---|---|
|  | Reproducer | |
|  | Boundary | |
| Ingestor | | Input transducer internal transducer |
| Distributor | | Channel and Net |
| Converter | | Decoder |
| Producer | | Associator |
| Matter-energy storage | | Memory |
|  | | Decider |
|  | | Encoder |
| Extruder | | Output transducer |
| Motor | | |
| Supporter | | |

produce, they generally fail to receive new inputs of matter-energy from their environments.

Besides pointing up some obvious difficulties, systems theory provides us with some potentially stimulating considerations. For example, Miller[5] has developed a number of hypotheses that help further relate the information processing subsystems to practical need assessment issues:

> There is always a constant systematic distortion between input and output of information in a channel.

In a channel there is always a progressive degradation of information and decrease in negative entropy or increase in noise or entropy. The output information per unit time is always less than it was at the input.

A system never completely compensates for the distortion in information flow in its channels.

A system tends to distort information in a direction to make it more likely to elicit rewards or less likely to elicit punishments to itself.

The less decoding and encoding a channel requires, the more it is used.

Over time a system tends to decrease the amount of recoding necessary within it, by developing more and more common systemwide codes.

Increase in the number of components in a system requires a disproportionately larger increase in the number of information processing and deciding components.

## Boundary Control

While some systems may be overly impervious to their environment, we must also concern ourselves with excessive boundary permeability. An organization too open to its environment can become overy reactive and lose the stability and continuity necessary for efficient production and growth. Information overload will produce organization and personal stresses due to the limited resources available to respond appropriately to all the information it has.

The issue of optimal boundary permeability is related to the necessity for systems to maintain a degree of stability or homeostasis. Too much instability produces system stress, increasing the rate of entropy. The issue can be examined in terms of overload or underload, of inputs or outputs, of matter-energy and/or information. Because human service agencies are primarily information-processing systems, we will restrict our analysis to the systemic effects of too much or too little information input and/or output.

Table 4–2 summarizes four basic conditions relating organi-

**Table 4–2    Four Conditions Arising From Organizational Action with Respect to Environmental Information**

| Organizational Action | Environmental Information | |
| --- | --- | --- |
| | Essential | Nonessential |
| 1. Permeable: Bring or allow in | Negentropy, effectiveness | Inefficiency, waste |
| 2. Impermeable: Filter or block out | Entropy, danger | Efficiency, saving |

zational action or reaction to environmental information. An organization may bring in too much nonessential information at considerable cost and inefficiency. More alarming is the case of filtering out or failing to bring in essential information. This situation will increase the inevitable process of entropy and may lead to a more acute disaster. It is never easy for managers to be precise in determining organization action because it is never clear what may be essential information. A third dimension could be added to this matrix, classifying the degree of environmental turbulence and uncertainty. As the latter increases, the organization will generally err in the direction of increased permeability. Frequently the manager may feel there is no choice, particularly when the environment, as exemplified by the community groups or government laws and regulations, forces information processing on the organization.

Systems initiate a variety of mechanisms to adjust to the stresses of information instability. Table 4–3 summarizes some of the major reactions to information overload and underload. Not all reactions can be considered adaptive. It is undoubtedly a sign of our times that we can think about a greater number of reactions to overload than we can for underload.

By comparison, some techniques, such as the nominal group approach or key informant survey, are based on the prior exist-

**Table 4–3    Systemic Reactions to Information Overload
and Information Underload**

| Information Overload | Information Underload |
|---|---|
| 1. Increase processing rates | 1. Increase environmental search |
| 2. Store inputs to process at slack time | 2. Decentralize information search |
| 3. Randomly omit some inputs | 3. Increase internal work processes |
| 4. Selectively filter | |
| 5. Abstract, consolidate, and generalize | 4. Increase fidelity of limited inputs |
| 6. Employ alternative channels | 5. Recycle old information |
| 7. Decentralize, delegate | 6. Ration information internally |
| 8. Forecast peak loads | 7. Dissolve (entropy) |
| 9. Escape | |
| 10. Explode (entropy) | |

ence of considerable information, or even information overload.
The need assessment process in these cases is equivalent to collecting a little more information to help organize, abstract, con-
solidate, or place in some perspectives of priorities and costs the
overwhelming amount of information the system already has.
Considered in this way, the choice of one or more needs assessment methodologies would be based, in part, on the system's
perception of information overload or underload.

## THE CITIZENS AND COMMUNITY AS SYSTEMS

Thus far, the emphasis has been on the importance of the
environmental monitoring process for agency adaptation and the
implications of systems theory for the methodology of need
assessment. Let us shift our perspective now to consider some
implications of systems theory for the purposes of the need
assessment process. Those who plan and conduct need assess-

ment studies may profit from viewing the citizen and the community as two other levels of systems.

By the premise that there are principles isomorphic to all levels of systems, we should expect principles that apply to organizational systems to apply as well to individuals. How do individuals adapt to information overload or underload? What are the effects of environmental change and uncertainty?

John Cassel,[12–14] a noted epidemiologist, makes some exciting suggestions regarding possible answers. After conducting his own research and reviewing the literature on animal and human illness, he suggests that the germ theory of disease is inadequate to explain the epidemiologic facts of major illnesses. Cassel makes a convincing argument that all disease, both "biologic" and "mental," is the result of a complex interaction of environmental agents (i.e., germs or toxins) and the general susceptibility of the organism. He argues that being placed in an environment where one's behavior no longer leads to predictable outcomes, or has an impact on that environment, raises one's generalized susceptibility to all types of disease or trauma. Whether one develops a disease will also depend on the social assets or support systems that the person has to buffer himself when placed within the turbulent and nonpredictable environment. In brief, Cassel indicates that the following four factors produce high stress and high levels of generalized susceptibility:

1. A high rate of environmental change.
2. A lack of predictability about the effects of change.
3. A lack of sufficient "turf control" or ability to influence the environment.
4. A lack of social supports or resources.

Germs are conceptualized as triggering agents of a disease process rather than as single causes of single effects. If we wish to prevent illness, Cassel suggests we reduce the general environmental conditions that lead to increased susceptibility.

Cassel's work suggests that environmental conditions will influence the person as a system in the same ways that environments influence organizations. But more important for our consideration here are the implications of the analysis for the type of need assessments we conduct.

Organizations responsible for a community need assessment should consider an assessment of those community groups or geographical areas most affected by environmental factors promoting stress and increased susceptibility. Instead of asking people about their specific problems, symptoms, or felt needs, we could be asking them such question as: How many changes have you recently experienced? How certain are you about your future living conditions? How much control do you feel you have over your own life circumstances? How many friends do you have? The answers could prove useful in predicting problems before they occur and in identifying areas with a high "need" for interventions designed to reduce the four negative environmental factors. Thus, we can apply the process of need assessment to the critical task of primary prevention.

What does general systems theory suggest for the need assessment process when we conceptualize the total community as the system? The agencies and citizens within the community now become system components that are more or less interconnected. An analysis of the community and the needs of its citizens would be comparable to an assessment of the internal allocation of the system's matter-energy to its internal components. In this case, it is important that the processes of internal transduction and decoding are sufficiently developed to allow for some standardized comparisons. Practically speaking, need assessment data would have to address broad ranges of human needs and human service resources. Interagency linkages (i.e., the channel and net) would have to be identified, and the flow of money, clients, staff, and information among agencies would have to be determined. This task is feasible if agencies have sufficiently developed MISs that allow for standardization of service definitions, staff time accounting procedures, client definition and identification, and fiscal record keeping. The assessment of citizen needs would have to be sensitive to common patterns of needs within single individuals. For example, studies by the Department of Health, Education, and Welfare indicate that as many as 86 to 95 percent of clients receiving a single categorical

HEW service have multiple problems.[15] Furthermore, the failure of the client to receive the proper mix of services is likely to render any single categorical service relatively ineffective when nudged by criteria of overall client functioning.

Data from a community-wide need assessment should have sufficient reliability and validity (i.e., information fidelity) to form the basis for decisions about the reallocation of scarce community resources. Presently, we lack much of the technology to achieve such fidelity. More critical, however, are the constraints imposed by the categorical nature of service planning, funding, and management. The federal government's service strategy of the 1950s and 1960s has created excessive fragmentation, duplication, discontinuity, inefficiency, and consequent ineffectiveness among the community service providers. The community as a system has become highly differentiated and poorly integrated. We know from systems theory that systems within complex environments must become highly differentiated. Subsystem differentiation promotes adaptation to complexity. Adaptive systems, however, also develop integrative mechanisms that hold the differentiated parts together.[11,16]

There are trends at all levels of government and service delivery to develop integrative mechanisms. Government reorganization, block grants, information and referral systems, integrated service networks, and health systems planning agencies are just a few examples of these attempts. The current legislative emphasis on need assessment also appears to be a response to the excessive specialization and fragmentation of the recent past.

Need assessors must think in terms of community systems and not use the process to justify further disintegration by promoting larger budgets for single categorical agencies. The need assessment process bears costs that must be justified in terms of its systemic contributions. Its justification must go beyond its legitimate use as a protective mechanism whereby agencies use "needs" data to garner larger budgets, more autonomy, and less accountability. Needs data must be collected that bears on resource allocation among agencies and on the gradual rates of impact of agency programs on community-wide problems. Furthermore, the need assessment process must begin to focus on what it can do to help prevent problems rather than treat them only after they have occurred and have been identified.

## Notes

1. Bertalanffy, L. von *General systems theory, foundations, development, applications*. New York: Braziller, 1968.

2. Buckley, W. (Ed.). *Modern systems research for the behavioral scientist*. Chicago: Aldine, 1968.

3. Emergy, R. E. (Ed.). *Systems thinking*. Baltimore: Penguin Books, 1969.

4. Miller, J. G. The nature of the living systems. *Behavioral Science*, 1971, *16*, 277–301.

5. Miller, J. G. Living systems: The organization. *Behavioral Science*, 1972, *17*, 1–182.

6. Baker, F. (Ed.) *Organizational systems: General systems approaches to complex organizations*. Homewood, Ill. Irwin, 1973.

7. Baker, F., Broskowski, A., & Brandwein, R. System dilemmas of a community health and welfare council. *The Social Service Review*, 1973, *47*, 63–79.

8. Katz, D., & Kahn R. *The social psychology of organizations*. New York: Wiley, 1966.

9. Wiener, N. *Cybernetics*. Cambridge, Mass.: Technology Press, 1948.

10. Ashby, W. R. *Design for a brain*. New York: Wiley, 1960.

11. Broskowski, A. Management information systems for planning and evaluation. In H. C. Schulberg & F. Baker (Eds.), *Program evaluation in the health fields* (Vol. II). New York: Behavioral Publications, 1976.

12. Cassel, J. C. Physical illness in response to stress. In S. Levine & N. Scotch (Eds.), *Social Stress*. Chicago: Aldine, 1970.

13. Cassel, J. C. Health consequences of population density and crowding. In National Academy of Sciences. *Rapid population growth*. Baltimore: Johns Hopkins Press, 1971.

14. Cassel, J. C. Psychiatric epidemiology. In G. Caplan (Ed.), *American handbook of psychiatry* (Vol. II). New York: Basic Books, 1973.

15. Department of Health, Education and Welfare. Interim report of the FY 1973 services integration R & D task force, 1973.

16. Lawrence, P., & Lorsch, J. Differentiation and integration in complex organizations. *Administrative Science Quarterly*, 1967, *12*, 1–47.

*Chapter 5*

# THE DEFINITION AND IDENTIFICATION OF HUMAN SERVICE NEEDS IN A COMMUNITY

*Tuan D. Nguyen,*
*C. Clifford Attkisson,*
*Marilyn J. Bottino*

With the emerging role of need assessment in human service program development, there is a sense of urgency to develop and refine assessment methods and strategies. The wide range of recently proposed techniques has stimulated many different definitions of "need." In consequence, persons with a common goal—need identification and assessment—may potentially work at cross purposes. Thus, it is a prerequisite to a meaningful discussion of approaches and methodologies to ask some crucial questions: Have advocates and researchers really defined their terms? If so, what consensus is there about the definition of need for health and human services?

## AN OVERVIEW OF APPROACHES TO AND PROBLEMS IN THE DEFINITION OF NEED

Our literature search reveals much conceptual and operational divergence regarding the definition of need for health and human service. This divergence applies both to the theoretical orientation underlying assessment strategies and the formal definition of need.

*Assumptions Underlying Needs Assessment Strategies*

Need assessment strategies have been well documented.[1,2] In the area of mental health and need assessment, Siegel, Attkisson, and Cohn[3] have identified the following types of information usually sought by each strategy or a combination thereof:[3]

1. Distribution of mental disorders in a population and factors influencing this distribution;
2. Relationships of social, health, or ecological characteristics of neighborhood or environment to rates of mental disorder;
3. Identification of the community's most urgent problems which command high priorities in terms of specific services to be developed;
4. Determination of the etiology of mental health disorder;
5. Identification of perspectives on the politics related to mental health in a community;
6. Identification of current and/or potential resources available for addressing identified problems;
7. Inventory of hospitalization and other service utilization rates.

The strategies for obtaining these types of information range from the simple use of service utilization statistics, through large-scale, sophisticatedly designed surveys, to community forums.[1,2] We think that, without undue oversimplification, the large number of assessment strategies available fall into one of three conceptual positions: rationalistic, empirical, and relativistic. This classification is not intended to be all-inclusive but rather is offered as a framework for thinking about needs assessment more concisely and critically.

*The Rationalistic Position.* From this perspective, need for health and human services is predicated on some pathology or deviance from a rationally determined ideal state of affairs. Two instrumentalities are usually employed to identify or anticipate divergence from ideal conditions: epidemiologic descriptors (symptoms and their prevalence or incidence) and sociodemographic indicators. Because both are highly technical, the responsibility for identifying and assessing needs for services lies with health and health-related professionals.

*The Empirical Position.* Empiricists conceive of need for health and human services as *deviance* from a normative or observed state of good health and well-being. They assume that such need motivates individuals to seek services and this need is translated into demand for services through the interplay of economic forces and the mechanisms of a free-market economy. According to the empiricist's position, specific assessment procedures beyond the study of demand for services are rarely required, although many empiricists have recently begun to analyze sociocultural factors that impede or facilitate the translation of wants and desires into demands.

*The Relativistic Position.* Relativists rely on the interplay of interest groups in the community to achieve a kind of sociocultural political consensus regarding the level and extent of need for services. They believe that comprehensive identification and assessment of needs must consider the full range of perspectives and values. Need assessors who embrace this position would like to:

1.  Gather the widest range of information on situations or circumstances that may qualify as need states.
2.  Submit this information to the widest range of interest groups for their considerations as to whether the situation or circumstance is a need state.
3.  Reconcile the diverse viewpoints regarding what needs actually exist at each level of social organization and how the services for meeting these identified needs should be rank-ordered in terms of their priorities.

Each of the three positions, rationalistic, empirical, and relativistic has strong points as well as shortcomings. The rationalistic position has strongly influenced the need assessment field. Its methodology is highly technical, and many currently favored strategies derive from it. However, statements about need based on these methodologies, because they are opinions of health and health-related professionals, represent a highly selected view-point. Similarly, statements about need derived from the empirical position, that is, based on indices of demand for services, are also limited because there are sociocultural factors that prevent conditions that can be interpreted as need states from being so recognized.[4] A need assessment program based on the relativistic position offers the possibility of the most comprehensive statements about health and human services needs at each level of community organization. However, it involves a complex process that has not been fully developed.

## Illustrative Definitions of Need

In addition to these three orientations, we also found a number of formal statements defining need. These definitions will now be reviewed as well as their implications for comprehensive need assessment.

Jeffers, Borganno, and Barlett,[5] after distinguishing between demand, want, and need for medical services, define need as:

> the quantity of medical services which medical opinion believes ought to be consumed (in order for the population) to remain or become as 'healthy' as is permitted by existing medical knowledge.

The definition may be extended to cover need for health and human service in general even though explicitly it addresses the question of need for medical services. It is important to note that the determination of need for services is contingent only upon medical opinion and existing medical knowledge. This definition does not allow input by the persons or groups whose needs are to be met or who may be affected by the implications of the assessment process.

A similar approach is offered by Saunder Lund:[6]

> When a circumstance is labeled necessary or desirable by those with control over the organization, a 'need' may be said to exist.

Presumably, the term *organization* refers to health and human service delivery systems and programs. Unlike Jeffers et al.,[5] Lund makes the determination of need for health and human service contingent upon the opinion of organizational control agents rather than medical experts. However, as Schaefer[7] has pointed out, "the information available to expert opinion is limited and perhaps imperfecty perceived." Moreover, even if technical information is perfect and available to everyone, the evaluation of that information will still not be unanimous or consistent among those drawing conclusions about the level and intensity of need for services.[7] Thus, one must question the wisdom of placing the burden and responsibility for determining need only on the shoulders of medical experts and control agents.

Wan and Soifer[8] are less restrictive concerning who is responsible for determining need:

> Need is usually measured by the symptoms of an illness
> perceived by the individual, his response and evaluation of
> the disabling effects, or by medical assessment of health
> status and physician rated urgency of the condition.

This conceptualization is strictly idiographic in that each instance of need is considered on an individual, case-by-case basis. For planning purposes, however, one must identify and assess need for services at all levels of social organization where health and human service delivery operations take place. Reiff[9] describes six strata of social organization: the individual, the group or family, the organization or social network, the institutional system, the community, and society. These are increasingly complex levels of social organization, each subsuming all the previous levels. A comprehensive need assessment program must identify needs at each level. Wan and Soifer's[8] definition that focuses only on needs at the level of the individual must be considered inadequate for such a program.

Blum, in his *Planning for Health*,[10] offers the most detailed approach to conceptualizing need for health services. In addition to elucidating the concepts of deviance, disability, illness, disease, and good health or well-being, he enumerates eight aspects of health which must be measured:

Prematurity of death
Disease
Discomfort or illness
Internal satisfaction
External satisfaction
Positive health
Capacity to participate

Blum[10] also enumerates indices for each aspect, at both individual and community levels. Presumably, when all aspects are measured, one would be in a position to plan effectively for health and human services. The difficulty, however, is that, as Blum himself put it: "Measurements define situations and attitudes convert situations into problems." Since the activity of measurement yields information, this information potentially can be converted into value-based statements of need. Determining the implications of these statements for social planning and program structure are yet further steps in this process.

Finally, Siegel, Attkisson and Cohn[3] view need as a relative concept, depending primarily upon those who undertake the identification and assessment effort. They define need as:

> the gap between what is viewed as a necessary level or condition by those responsible for this determination and what actually exists.

This relativistic approach is congruent with the present state of affairs in which need assessments are by and large activities that are unrelated to one another. However, it fails to sow the seed for the development of a more integrative approach.

In summary, our examination of approaches to measuring and defining need for health and human service lead us to identify the following four conceptual and operational deficiencies:

1.  Exclusive reliance on expert opinion or organizational control agents for determining when a need state exists.

2. Insufficient emphasis on and lack of consideration for need states that transcend the individual level of social organization.
3. Lack of specific operational criteria for determining the existence of a need state and for differentiating between met and unmet needs.
4. Lack of a systematic framework with which to integrate divergent methodologic inputs into the process of need identification and assessment.

## Issues and Problems in Conceptualizing Need

In addition to the above list of deficiencies, there are also five crucial issues that must be resolved prior to achieving comprehensive need assessment.

First, how dependent should a conceptualization of need be on measurement strategies? This is the issue of the line of development between theory or conceptualization on the one hand and method or measurement on the other.[11] A short line of development exists when a concept is tied extremely closely to the method used to validate it, for example, when intelligence is defined as "what the I.Q. test says it is." While often thought to foster scientific parsimony, it often shifts the focus away from the validation process, narrowing the attention to the instruments or apparatus used. In terms of need identification and assessment, a short line of measurement may eventuate in polemical debates concerning the merits and superiorities of measuring instruments without much constructive results for program planning and evaluation. Even if one strategy is voted as the method of choice, premature adherence to it can thwart creativity and resourcefulness in our approach to need identification and assessment.[12] Creativity and resourcefulness are culturally based on the premises that a free flow of ideas and open competition generally result in the most innovative and resourceful programs or methodologies being those that are implemented. Can it then follow that this approach be predicated solely on the mechanisms of a free-market economy? The free-market economy model, as applied to health and human service planning, assumes that needs for services are accurately expressed as demand for services, presumably measurable by admissions to existing service facilities. This model is not applicable to health and human service delivery because of conceptual and operational difficulties related to the use of expressed demand as an approach to need assessment.[13]

> In counting admissions, what is to be considered a "case"?
>
> Institutions differ in their practices regarding what type of contact for service qualifies as an admission and what does not.
>
> Admission rates may be misleading because of duplicated counts resulting from a single individual having multiple admissions during a given period to a single institution and its service components or to different institutions.
>
> What constitutes a health and human service facility, for example, a mental health facility, is defined differently from one geographical area to another.
>
> Needers of health and human services are not always utilizers, and the utilizers of these services may not be persons who need it most.[14]

In short, to define and identify need solely on the basis of demand for services is to take a narrow conceptual approach.

Second, are all need states directly observable? What are the implications for the science of need assessment if some need states are directly observable and measurable while others remain inferred. And what are the implications of focusing assessment only on directly observable and measurable need states?

These problems are not idiosyncratic to the social sciences. For example, in high-energy physics, while the psi particle cannot be measured directly, its properties can be ascertained with reasonable accuracy and certainty based on the antecedent and consequent manifestations of its occurrence. Similarly, certain need states may not be directly observed but can be predicted by observing their antecedent or predisposing conditions and inferred as "real" on the basis of their consequences.

Third, even if a need state is directly observable and measurable, do all observers necessarily agree upon its implications for

program planning and program development? Inputs into the
conceptualization and perception of need come from varied
sources with particular perspectives that may or may not be
congruent or commensurate with each other.[1] Each perspective,
nonetheless, must be considered to be a valid perceptual filter
revealing one view of the social situation. There is, then, ground
for questioning any attempt to establish a monolithic oligarchy
predicated on any single perspective and /or measurement
method.

Fourth, since the value systems and cultural configuration in
a community do not remain static, how can a health and human
service delivery system respond to the flux and influx of changing needs and priorities? Need identification and assessment are
in a sense a monitoring of the environmental context surrounding a health and human service delivery system.[15] As Blum[10] has
pointed out, assessment is a signal system that:

> Provides . . . early warning signals of current deficits, sur-
> pluses, use and misuse of health resources;
> Offers clues, suggests intervention and, ultimately, helps to
> develop means of verifying the etiology and the predispos-
> ing or aggravating factors in various conditions which need
> to be subjected to medical and ecological research;
> Uncovers discrepancies which signal failures of prediction
> or of reasoning about the influences acting on well-being:
> (Identifies) the boundaries which are relevant for successful
> attack on a given condition;
> Provides information about community value systems, and
> about political, social, and economic outlooks (which are
> useful to planning bodies for deciding) where to start health
> and human service planning and when the conditions are
> ripe for action.

Given Blum's systemic functions of need assessment, need
assessors and researchers must face the crucial issue of how to
conceptualize need so that they can achieve the desired goal of
producing an early warning system. Figure 5–1 presents a sche-
ma of the interrelationship between needs and services. In any
community there exist needs (delimited by the circle), some identified and some unrecognized. Among the identified needs, some

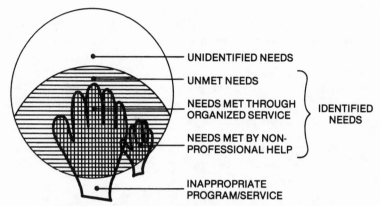

**Figure 5–1 Relationship between needs and service programs**

are met through organized, programmatic efforts (large hand) or through informal help (small hand), but many are still not met in any manner (unmet needs). Need assessment should specifically address the needs that are heretofore unrecognized and needs that have not been met.

The final issue concerns the proper focus of need assessment. Should it deal only with individual needs? If not, what are the levels of community and social organization where needs are to be assessed? In some definitions of need, we found a sharp focus on the individual; in others, we detected an emphasis on some higher level of social organization; in still others, there was no specification as to the level where need is to be identified.

As previously noted, Rieff[9] has described six levels of social organization, each subsuming all the prior levels. However, needs that exist at a lower level may not be generalizable to higher levels, and each level may also have needs that are not salient to another level. For example, at the individual level, there are needs for personal well-being and health. At the level of the family, needs may relate to concerns for the integrity of kinship ties and economic stability, in addition to concerns for the health and well-being of family members. At the community level, attention may be focused primarily on preserving the geographical and political identity and social values of the community. Thus, given the differences in content and nature between needs that exist at different levels of social organization, any conceptualization that focuses only on one level will prove inadequate for comprehensive needs assessment.

Up to this point we have reviewed and evaluated existing conceptual approaches and definitions of need as well as examined crucial issues in comprehensive needs assessment. The following points can be summarized regarding the prerequisites to an adequate conceptualization of need;

> Need must not be defined solely in terms of the method or strategy used to measure its antecedent or consequent conditions.
>
> Need can be an inferred state of affairs. While its occurrence is predictable on the basis of certain conditions, it is not always directly observable.
>
> Inputs into the conceptualization and the perception of need come from many perspectives. Need, therefore, is a relative concept, and community agreement about priorities among needs is a prerequisite to taking action on the information about needs.
>
> The assessment of need is productive insofar as it functions as an environmental monitoring system to provide early warnings for health and human service programs and helps identify unrecognized or unmet needs.
>
> Needs at one level of social organization do not necessarily reflect those at a different level. Consequently, a comprehensive need assessment must document and assess needs at each level of social organization.

We believe that it is possible to conceptualize need such that all of the above points are met. In light of our earlier discussion regarding met and unmet needs (see also Fig. 1), it seems appropriate to focus our attention on needs that are either unmet or unrecognized.

## DEFINITION OF UNMET NEED

An unmet need is said to exist when certain conditions prevail:

1.  The recognition of a problem, a dysfunctional somatic or psychological state, or an undesirable social process.
2.  The judgment that possible satisfactory solutions are not accessible, are not currently adequate, or do not exist in the community.
3.  The necessity to reallocate existing resources and/or appropriate new resources.

"Problem" refers to the perceived discrepancy between what exists and what is deemed desirable or necessary. Problem areas include dysfunctional somatic, psychological, physical, social, or economic conditions. The perception of discrepancy involves a judgment about how a given situation or circumstance compares with an ideal. In other words, the concept "problem" involves: (1) a perception of what is, (2) a comparison level, i.e., what should be, and (3) an evaluation of the extent and saliency of the discrepancy between the two. The ideal may be defined explicitly, or it may exist only implicitly in the mind of the person who perceives the discrepancy. In either case, values, tastes, preferences, and attitudes play an important role in defining this ideal condition. Blum has illustrated this point as follows:[10]

> Enumerations are, of course, conceptually premeditated and thereby produce so-called facts. These facts are believed to identify conditions or situations. What is perceived is a condition which is not necessarily good or bad per se. The identical situation may be seen as good by those whose value expectations are met, and bad by those whose values are not; those whose values are unrelated, or who do not connect the condition to values, may not perceive the condition at all, or view it as a neutral state of affairs. The situation may be seen as different things by those who hold different concepts of the system of which it is a part.

"Recognition of a problem" refers to the process of determining the discrepancy between what exists and what is deemed desirable or necessery. Who, then, recognizes the problem? Our answer is "Whoever participates in or is responsible for need assessment." This means concerned citizens, interest and political groups, consumers of health and human services, funders, program planners, service providers, as well as health and health-related professionals. If problem recognition is not the exclusive prerogative of a specific agent or group, what then is the proper method for this recognition? We do not consider it feasible or proper to impose a prescribed method. To require that everyone uses, for example, the epidemiologic approach or the service utilization approach is to restrict a priori the process of problem recognition to a given perspective on the situation to be assessed. However, we are not resigned to eclecticism, for we do believe that there is a process whereby concensus can be reached regarding needs and their priorities. This process will be discussed in greater detail in our presentation of the convergent analysis approach to comprehensive need assessment. The gist of this approach is the conviction that;

1. Need identification must be achieved through a wide range of methodologies and strategies.
2. The identified information must be integrated in a progressive, sequential manner.
3. The above is necessary to achieve a kind of sociocultural and political consensus regarding needs for health and human services.

"Satisfactory solutions" refer to the activities, programs, or services viewed as capable of reducing the gap between what actually exists and what is deemed desirable or necessary. Values and attitudes again play a predominant role. A satisfactory, desirable, or necessary solution for one group may not be acceptable to another. Furthermore, there is not a necessary isomorphism, that is, one-to-one relationship, between the problem and its solution regarding either their intrinsic natures or the levels of social organization where they occur. For example, individual problems such as alienation may be resolved by actions taken at the group, family, or community level. As another example, economic interventions are sometimes the only meaningful solutions to undesirable social problems.

Problem recognition and solution identification occur within the systems of values, preferences, and attitudes of persons within the community that undertakes need assessment. But if persons undertaking these activities do not hold similar values and attitudes, how will they reach consensus regarding what situations represent the most pressing need states among those that are identified?

We propose resource assessment as the key process in arriving at consensus about the relative priorities among unmet needs. Resource refers, in the most general sense, to the means of achieving the desired remediation of unmet needs. Because money is a common denominator in economic exchange, often it is defined in terms of financial resources. However, resources include also technical knowledge, professional expertise in solving problems, the time and effort available for achieving solutions, as well as other intangible assets such as the emotional support and empathy provided to those in need.

Solutions to problems require the expenditure or mobilization of resources. Even programs that use volunteer services involve time and effort on the part of professional staff to train volunteers and on the part of volunteers to deliver the services. Funds are also necessary to sustain even a minimum organizational structure in these programs and to secure necessary materials. Need assessment should, then, provide planners with information on how much, and whether, resources should be expended in a given area of concern. Need assessment should also serve to justify the investment of resources in programs. A need assessment program that does not produce results for decision making and planning will remain a vacuous enterprise.

We believe that the proper focus of need assessment should embrace all levels of social organization. At the individual level, problems often arise because the person's role in the economic system proves unsatisfactory, goals of personal well-being and health are not met, social interactions are grossly dysfunctional, or the individual's ecologic environment has been drastically disturbed. Each area of functioning, singly or in combination with another, can give rise to a specific problem in living or need state. Given the wide range of problems and their interrelationships that affect the individual, a narrow focus often results in the promotion of categorical programs or services that fail to consider the total person.

At the higher end of the spectrum of social organization, that is, the community level, the value system and the social-political structure of the commonwealth as a whole, when dysfunctional, can also give rise to problems. In addition to humanitarian concerns, the community values the freedom and equal rights of its members, their security, and the long range development of opportunities. Solutions are satisfactory to the extent that they respect or help foster the realization of these valued goals. But they must also be examined in terms of the burden placed on the economic and human resources of the community.

In summary, our definition of need implies a sequential process of determining and documenting:

1.  The need situation for each level of social organization, in light of the values, tastes, preferences, attitudes, and the existent knowledge in the community.
2.  The resources required to narrow the discrepancy between what is and what should be.
3.  The consensus regarding relative priorities of unmet needs.
4.  The programmatic deployment of resources.

## CONVERGENT ANALYSIS

Our conceptualization of need implies three goals to be achieved in comprehensive need assessment.

1.  First, needs must be assessed at all levels of social organization.
2.  Second, need assessment must have relevance for the planning of services and programs.
3.  Finally, but not least importantly, the widest range of information must be brought to bear on the process of assessing needs.

How then does one achieve these three goals? What is the method or strategy for reaching them? We believe that the goals of comprehensive need assessment as outlined above can be achieved by applying the concept of convergent analysis to need assessment.[1]

Convergent analysis is a methodologic and conceptual framework in which information relative to human service needs is assessed and given priority in a progressive, sequential manner. It is the second of two operational stages in establishing the need states in a social area, the other being need identification.

In the need identification stage, the primary task is to collect the widest range of information using need documentation methods. The synthesis and integration of this information is accomplished through convergent analysis.[1]

> Convergent analysis usually begins with data that are internal to the service system, such as legal and funder mandates, historical trends relevant to service delivery, and client utilization information. This is the store of data that need assessment often shares with evaluation. But, in addition to it, there is information about the orientation, training and interests of administrators and providers, and the perspectives of advisory and policy board members as well as the viewpoints of citizens. The process then integrates information assembled about a specified social area or target community via a network of techniques designed to capture a wide range of perceptions about conditions in the community.

As stated previously, need assessment is best viewed as consisting of two phases: (1) problem recognition and (2) solution identification through convergent analysis. In the first phase, one attempts to explore and identify areas where there are discrepancies between existing and desired or necessary conditions. The methodologies involved range from community surveys, through socioeconomic indicator analysis, to community group approaches.[1]

In the second phase of solution identification, one attempts to accomplish three tasks: (1) integrate the wide range of data and perspectives collected; (2) explore the nature of the solutions to identified problems; and (3) identify the types and levels of resources necessary for these solutions. The third task is necessary because the intensity and extent of need depend not only on the intensity and extent of problems, but also on the amount and type of resources that must be deployed to solve the problems. Often, a problem is perceived on the basis of incomplete information. A problem may also arise when existing solutions are perceived as inadequate or unsatisfactory. The interchange of information and perceptions among interested parties and the negotiation among these parties concerning resource mobilization or redeployment can lead to consensus regarding needs and problematic situations.

Convergent analysis involves several presuppositions:

1. No single need documentation technique and no single set of stakeholders can offer a comprehensive view of the human service needs in a particular community.
2. Each technique portrays an aspect of the existing reality and provides important, though necessarily limited, clues about need states and the populations in our communities most likely to suffer from them.
3. The process of synthesizing these separate views allows a reasonably viable portrait of the problems in the community under study.

In sum, following Siegel, Attkisson, and Carson:[1]

> Convergent analysis is used here in the sense that the integrated sum of a series of measuring tools, deployed both systematically and sequentially, will yield a reasonably accurate identification of community needs and an assessment of the relative priorities of the needs identified.

Three additional conceptual issues further define the meaning of convergent analysis as Siegel, Attkisson and Carson see it:[1]

1. First, there is a convergence of different information coming from divergent viewpoints concerning needs for services (e.g., citizens, consumers, service providers, political leaders).
2. Second, there is a convergence of different assessment strategies, each with some overlapping, yet unique bits of information.

3.  Third, convergent also describes the cumulative nature
    of an ideal assessment procedure viewed across time.

All three of the above conceptualizations of convergent
analysis imply that, with each step-wise increment in information
from a wider range of methods and a wider range of perspectives,
one more clearly approximates a valid description of the social
area under study. Convergent analysis, then, provides a dynamic
process for reaching a convergent and discriminant validation of
the needs in a social area.

As we read the relevant literature, it is clear that the first
stage of need assessment, that is, need determination, has received a large share of attention and therefore is much more fully
developed than the second state. Much remains then to be done
to develop methodologies that are both crucial to and congruent
with convergent analysis. We believe that when such methodologies are developed and refined, need assessors will be better able
to embark on comprehensive need assessment.

In developing methodologies for collecting, analyzing, and
integrating data relevant to need assessment, however, much
effort can be saved if one examines the interrelationship of need
assessment with another informational system in health and human service programs: program evaluation. Many methodologies inherent to program evaluation may be applicable to need
assessment to the extent that the two informational systems contribute to program planning and development.

## LINKAGE BETWEEN NEED ASSESSMENT AND PROGRAM EVALUATION

Before discussing the methodologic and functional relationships between need assessment and program evaluation, we
want to emphasize that need assessment is conceptually separate
and operationally different from program evaluation. Need
assessment must not be confused with or subsumed as a subset of
program evaluation.

Attkisson and Broskowski[16] have defined program evaluation as:

The process of making reasonable judgments about program effort, effectiveness, efficiency, and adequacy.

Based on systematic data collection and analysis.

Designed for use in program management, external accountability, and future planning.

With special focus on accessibility, acceptability, awareness, availability, comprehensiveness, continuity, integration, and cost of services.

Need assessment, by contrast, is:

An environmental monitoring system.

Designed to measure and make judgments about program relevance, adequacy, and appropriateness

Based on systematic collection and analysis of information

Regarding the needs for health and human services

As filtered through multiple levels of societal perspectives.

As generated through multiple measurement approaches.

In other words, need assessment studies monitor social area and population characteristics that influence need, want, and demand for human services. These factors include the value systems and ethnocultural backgrounds of the population being served. Especially important are the analyses of cultural, psychological, physical, environmental, and linguistic barriers to appropriate service utilization. Need assessment analyses therefore must focus on issues related to population characteristics, environmental characteristics, individual citizen need states, as well as five other critical issues related to the overall effectiveness and appropriateness of the total service delivery system:[16]

Availability of services relative to population characteristics.

Accessibility of services relative to populaton need states, environmental characteristics, and distribution of service resources.

Awareness of service opportunities among the residents of the social area.

Level of service integration and continuity of services vis-a-vis multiproblem individuals and the availability of service network linkages.

Level of resources and distribution of available resources vis-a-vis need states in the social area.

Put differently, need assessment data provide a fundamental navigational system for program planning and modification based on continuous assessment of changing community needs. Without need assessment input, health and human service programs stand little change to "weather the storms" resulting from the pressures of vested interests, bureaucracy, and professionally defined needs.

Information from program evaluation, on the other hand, is an internal monitoring system that assesses the achievement of the programs in terms of goals and mandates. Without input from program evaluation, health and human services will continue to be managed without benefit of critical information about program effort, efficiency, and effectiveness.

Both need assessment and program evaluation are thus crucial to the survival, growth, and structural soundness of health and human service programs.[1]

> Through analysis of program inputs, throughputs, and outputs, program evaluation allows judgments about whether program aspirations materialized at the cost, to the degree, in the manner specified, and a determination of whether the program remains relevant in terms of cost-effectiveness in dealing with services demanded and provided. In program evaluation, movement is measured toward or away from a predefined and expected level of output due to specified interventions; whereas need assessment is aimed at gathering environmental baseline information for purposes of establishing whether program resources are targeted at domains of greatest need relevance in a given social area.

Within health and human service programs, there must be a clear and open interface between the need assessment and program evaluation data collection and analysis systems. This interface requires specific collaboration and integration of these two program planning systems to avoid redundant activity, particularly where there is a clear overlap in data collection and analysis.

The overlapping responsibility is particularly clear in the analyses of:

> Service acceptability.
> Service accessibility.
> Demand for specific services.
> Continuity of services.
> Comprehensiveness of services.
> Pattern of service utilization.
> Resource availability.
> Resource utilization.

Program evaluation and need assessment are, consequently, significantly interdependent processes. Each consumes information from the other and provides an information base essential for program planning. Planners need both sets of information, and their work will be deficient unless both are simultaneously available. As Attkisson and Broskowski point out:[16]

> Programs can be internally consistent and relevant, can be cost-efficient and produce excellent cost-outcomes without necessarily being externally relevant, or represent the most efficient use of the total resource pool. An internally consistent and cost-efficient program does not necessarily produce satisfactory deployment of resources given the need state distribution of the social area served by the human service program.
>
> Program evaluation information made available without sensitive environmental monitoring of needs can actually undermine the program planning process. Without knowledge of needs, plans for program continuance are made vacuously outside of a meaningful context for decision making.
>
> The current categorical approach to service delivery delimits the systemic effectiveness of our overall human service network. As program evaluation methodology improves, this low level of effectiveness will increasingly become apparent. Efforts to improve the integration of the current categorical

system through a system of linkages and administrative efficiencies are needed if we are to enhance the effectiveness of the currently poorly integrated matrix of categorical services.

## Notes

1. Siegel, L. M., Attkisson, C. C., & Carson, L. G. Need identification and program planning in the community context. In C. C. Attkisson, W. A. Hargreaves, M. J. Horowitz, & J. E Sorensen (Eds.), *Evaluation of human service programs.* New York: Academic Press, 1978.

2. Warheit, G. J., Bell, R. A., & Schwab, J. J. *Planning for change: Needs assessment approaches.* Rockville, Md.: National Institute of Mental Health, 1974.

3. Siegel, L. M., Attkisson, C. C., & Cohn, A. H. Mental health needs assessment: Strategies and techniques. In W. A. Hargreaves, C. C. Attkisson, L. M. Siegel, M. H. McIntyre, & J. E. Sorensen (Eds.), *Resource materials for community mental health program evaluation* (Part III). Rockville, Md.: National Institute of Mental Health, 1974.

4. Wan, T. T. H., & Soifer, S. J. A multivariate analysis of the determinants of physician utilization. *Journal of Socio-economic Planning Sciences,* 1975, *390,* 1–9.

5. Jeffers, J. R., Borganno, M. F., & Bartlett, J. C. On the demand versus need for medical services and the concept of "shortage." *American Journal of Public Health,* 1971, *61,* 46–63.

6. Lund, S. The role of goal attainment scaling in a goal-oriented evaluation system: One man's view. *Program Evaluation Project Newsletter,* Vol. IV, 6, July–August, 1973. Hennepin County Program Evaluation Project, Minneapolis, Minnesota.

7. Schaefer, M. E. Demand versus need for medical services in a general cost-benefit setting. *Public Health Briefs,* 1975, *20,* 293–295.

8. Wan, T. T. H., & Soifer, S. J. Determinants of physician utilization: A causal analysis. *Journal of Health and Social Behavior,* 1974, *15,* 100–108.

9. Attkisson, C. C., McIntyre, M. H., Hargreaves, W. A., Harris, M.

R., & Ochberg, F. M. A working model for mental health program evaluation. *American Journal of Orthopsychiatry*, 1974, *44*(5), 741–753.

10. Blum, H. L. *Planning for health*. New York: Human Services Press, 1974, pp. 165–185, 213–220, 227.

11. Rychlak, J. F. *A philosophy of science for personality theory*. Boston: Houghton Mifflin, 1968, pp. 215–220.

12. Schulberg, H. C., & Wechsler, H. The uses and misuses of data in assessing mental health needs. *Community Mental Health Journal*, 1967, *3*, 389–395.

13. Henisz, J. E., Tischler, G. L., & Myers, J. K. Epidemiologic and ecologic analyses. In D. C. Reidel, J. K. Myers, & G. T. Tischler (Eds.), *Patient care evaluation in mental health programs*. Cambridge, Massachusetts: Ballinger, 1974, pp. 53–54.

14. Schwab, J. J., Warheit, G. J. & Fennell, E. B. *Community mental health evaluation: An assessment of needs and services*, 1973. (unpublished).

15. Broskowski, A., & Driscoll, J. How to think about organizations: Classic and systemic theories. In C. C. Attkisson, W. A. Hargreaves, M. J. Horowitz, & J. E. Sorensen (Eds.), *Evaluation of human service programs*. New York: Academic Press, 1978.

16. Attkisson, C. C., & Broskowski, A. Evaluation and the emerging human service concept. In C. C. Attkisson, W. A. Hargreaves, M. J. Horowitz, & J. E. Sorensen (Eds.), *Evaluation of human service programs*. New York: Academic Press, 1978.

*Chapter 6*

# THE MEASUREMENT OF HEALTH STATUS

## Danielle M. Turns,
## Larry G. Newby

Our attempts to define and measure health remind one of Freud's repetition-compulsion concept, "that is the blind impulse to repeat earlier experiences and situations quite irrespective of any advantage that doing so might bring from a pleasure-pain point of view."[1] Not only do we lack consensus on an operational or theoretical definition of health, but we keep trying to measure this undefined condition by its absence. This has brought much pain and little pleasure.

Social scientists have been unable to attain consensus on a definition of health that is applicable in all situations. The World Health Organization defined it as a "state of complete physical, mental and social well-being and not merely the absence of disease or infirmity."[2] Such an abstract definition has a number of empirical as well as theoretical limitations. The major theoretical complaints are: (1) mental and social well-being are compatible with some degree of disease or infirmity; (2) it is highly unlikely there ever is, or could be, more than a transient state of complete health for individuals or societies; and (3) practitioners do not necessarily need to know what constitutes health to treat patients.[3] This conceptualization has been both applauded and criticized for equating well-being with health. But, is the euphoric manic healthy? Is the wholehearted Nazi in a pro-Nazi society healthy? Furthermore, the definition expresses an ideal state rather than identifying particular conditions in man. Hence, it has a certain static quality that does not account for life fluctuations.

As Dubos said:[4]

> Life is an adventure in a world where nothing is static . . . The very process of living is a continual interplay between the individual and his environment, often taking the form of a struggle resulting in disease or injury . . . In reality, complete freedom from disease and struggle is almost incompatible with the process of living.

Sir Aubrey Lewis' definition emphasizes the relativity of health: "The terms health and illness are useful fictions which refer to uplands and lowlands in a gradually graded and terraced country."[5] These statements, both true and poetic, epitomize the quandary of the health epidemiologist.

Apart from the theoretical difficulties with the WHO definition, measurement difficulties abound since a single index will not reflect the full range of meanings associated with the nature and extent of health. Sullivan states that classifying individuals by established criteria of health is "meaningful only within an implicit or explicit frame of reference."[6] Such a frame of reference for classification would include the purpose, the observation rules, and the assumption that observations can be made. Utility of measure is a primary consideration in selecting indicators of the characteristics of persons or populations. Such indicators serve to bound the measure within certain limits. In short, health as defined by WHO is merely a verbal artifact and becomes useful as a measurement tool only within the confines of specific criteria. Since health can be defined narrowly or broadly, measurement precision will vary accordingly.

None of the many other existing definitions are satisfactory from either an operational or conceptual point of view. The qualifications of health as "undisturbed rhythm,"[7] "optimal personal fitness,"[8] "perfect continuing adjustment,"[9] or "reasonably free from undue pain"[10] use words which themselves have different meanings in different contexts. Dorn has attempted to define and measure health more rigorously.[11] In his discussion of data-gathering methods, he postulates three central criteria for establishing ill health: (1) individual's self perception, (2) clinical examination, and (3) diagnostic tests. Sullivan advances these criteria by proposing specific indicators of subjective and clinical evidence and includes other indicators, which he calls behavioral evidence.[6] Absenteeism, functional restrictions, medical expenditures, utilization and institutionalization statistics, and role loss would be examples of behavioral evidence of illness. Elinson outlines six currently used measures of morbidity.[12] Three are used by social scientists (in contrast to medical clinicians) in measuring illness: self-reports of symptoms, others' observations of signs of illness, and reports of cognitive awareness not readily observable. However, because of the "dynamic nature of health and disease, it is not likely that an index of health . . . will satisfy all (users) from the standpoint of . . . needs."[13]

To date we have not adequately defined health. Have we done better in measuring its absence? Traditional measures of the health status of a population include mortality and morbidity rates. Death is by and large a well defined and recorded event that, until recently, has been considered valid. As to morbidity, precise operational definitions of a condition would enable an investigator to distinguish between "cases" and "normals." But clear-cut transitions from illness to health or from one type of morbidity to another are the exception rather than the rule. We do not have criteria for establishing the absence of all conditions in one person, and we may never finish enumerating all the cases because we never finish defining the mildest varieties.

### PROBLEMS IN MEASURING HEALTH STATUS

These difficulties in conceptualizing health and disease are perhaps the major constraints on the development and usefulness of health status indicators. We will briefly describe the most commonly used indicators and examine their inherent problems: validity (does the instrument measure what is supposedly being measured?), reliability (that is, the consistency with which it measures it), data sources, and cost.

## Mortality Data Base

As previously stated, mortality rates (including infant or maternal mortality) have been useful for measuring the health status of populations and for comparing populations. However, not only is the reliability of infant mortality data, for example, still in question, but it has also been demonstrated that it "appears to no longer be a particularly useful indicator of the level of living and sanitary conditions for a country like the United States."[13] This is because the United States is more heterogeneous than most developed or underdeveloped nations. An index that averages the mortality of the best served groups who have low birth rates with that of the least served groups with high birth rates is not a satisfactory reflection of reality.

When mortality data is analyzed in terms of specific conditions, its reliability is again open to question. One significant hurdle is that only one cause of death may be recorded, whereas many other conditions existing at the time of death are ignored in a routine statistical approach. Even when there is only one obvious cause, the recording may be distorted. For example, it is well known that the recording of suicide as a particular cause of death is erratic as cultural attitudes toward suicide are reflected in coroners' or medical examiners' practices.[14] The recording is also influenced by considerations such as the individual's social status, whether or not there is an insurance policy with a suicide exclusion clause, etc. Another example of distorted recording is the age-specific death rates given for cancer.[15] For most cancers, the mortality rates increase linearly with age; however, this trend usually reverses itself in age groups over 75 years. It is true that because of the smaller population base involved the rates are not stable, but there should be no reason for statistical variability to express itself consistently in a downward trend beyond the age of 75 years. Another explanation may be that people who are blessed with longevity just do not get cancer. Still another possibility, at least for lung cancer mortality, is that people born long before the smoking epidemic were not as likely to be exposed to the carcinogen and truly have lower rates. But another probable explanation is that the cause of death in the very old is not investigated in the same manner as for younger age groups. Cancer in the very old is usually slow-growing and may not manifest many symptoms. Whatever symptoms it creates may be lost among those due to other pathology. Furthermore, the death of a 90-year-old person is likely to be attributed to old age, and a clinically unidentified disease is not likely to be recorded as cause of death.

## Morbidity Data Base

Another widely used series of health statistics are treated morbidity and facility utilization rates. We earlier touched upon the difficulties associated with various definitions of illness. What we will concentrate upon now are the distortions introduced by the treated rates. The gist of the matter is that entry in treatment is influenced by factors that have little to do with the presence of illness.

First, at least for mental disorders, the distance between a treatment facility and the community it serves is a powerful determinant of admission rates; the farther the facility, the lower the admission rate.[16] For tuberculosis, the Saranac Lake syndrome is well-known to epidemiologists: the presence of specialized centers of good reputation induces a selective migration of patients with the particular disease.

Second, economic factors may be severe obstacles. The lower middle class, with minimal insurance coverage, may not seek treatment for a condition which would send a welfare or an upper class individual to a clinic or a physician, and the morbidity goes unrecorded.[17]

Third, communities' attitudes toward health facilities, particularly in underdeveloped countries, are crucial in care-seeking. It is not unusual to see a brand new facility with modern equipment go practically unused. There is enough pathology around, but because of cultural superstitions or bad public relations, or both, the people do not utilize these facilities. Obviously, relying on utilization rates in such cases will not give an accurate reflection of morbidity.

Fourth, treatment facilities can affect their utilization rates by administrative policies. This was done in England where the revolving door policy reduced mental hospitals' populations prior to the introduction of the neuroleptics.[18] Also, this phenomenon was observed in New York State where restrictions on admissions of the elderly led to a drastic drop in their admission rates.[19] Neither the drop in census nor the decrease in the elderly's admissions reflected a true change in the incidence or prevalence of mental disorders in those groups.

Administrative policies may also wipe out entire disease entities in one clean sweep. One of the best illustrations is the story of the Chief of the French Armed Forces during World War I. Upset because of the soaring rates of gonorrhea among the French soldiers, he called his surgeon general and in no uncertain terms expressed his displeasure. The poor surgeon was torturing himself trying to find a solution when a bulb lit up. He sent a memo to all army physicians ordering that, as of immediately, all new cases of gonorrhea would be called "urethral discharge of unknown etiology." Gonorrhea was the French's first defeated enemy in that war! In short, treated morbidity is the tip of the iceberg, and that tip is crooked; some social groups are overrepresented, and some are underrepresented, as to the true morbidity of the population.

Fifth, another category of difficulties involves case duplication. It is not unusual for a person with one disease entity to have several simultaneously and to be using a variety of facilities at the same time. Nor is it unusual for a person with one condition to frequent several facilities. When attempts are made to identify which groups have higher morbidity rates than others, the characteristics of those multiple users are given undue weight.

Last but not least, a major obstacle in estimates based on treated morbidity or utilization rate is the problem of under- versus overutilization. Possibly a term better than overutilization is "misutilization." People who are heavy users of given facilities are not necessarily overutilizing them, but in all likelihood they are going to the wrong ones. For example, the hypochondriac who goes to several different clinics may be better off going to only one: the mental health center. The fallacy that segments of the population should be proportionately represented in utilization patterns is still around. Yet we maintain, and many have said it better, the fact that 25 percent of our population consists of children does not mean that 25 percent of persons receiving care should be children. The elderly represent only about 15 percent of our population, but many of their health needs are much greater than those of children and most adults.

It is imperative to determine the influence of subjective states upon utilization behavior. A review of the literature illustrates the emergence of several alternative patterns.[20,21] Without underrating the other research findings, three themes appear to be dominant: (1) the seriousness of the illness is a primary factor in explaining the frequency, type, and nature of services utilized; (2) differentials in the prevalence rates of services' utilization may be largely accounted for by unequal access that can be minimized, particularly by reducing economic barriers; and (3) sociocultural factors, especially the lay referral structure, are important determinants of utilization behavior.[22]

It should be kept in mind that information derived from treated cases may give a fallacious idea of the general expected outcome of a specific disorder. Prior to the discovery of streptomycin, pulmonary tuberculosis was seen as a killer disease because (1) the more severe cases were in treatment, and (2) some of the treatments were harmful. But many an ambulatory untreated TB patient had spontaneous remissions.

## COMMUNITY SURVEYS AND HEALTH STATUS DETERMINATION

Let us now examine the pitfalls in the measurement of morbidity derived from community surveys. The National Health Survey gathered a wealth of data on the population's acute and chronic conditions, days lost from work or school, activities' limitations, etc.[23] In spite of the great care used in training interviewers and the sophisticated analysis techniques, reliability checks have shown that the accuracy of respondent reports depend on (1) the type of illness, (2) the socioeconomic status of the respondent, (3) the length of hospitalization, and (4) the time elapsed. Surveys besides self-reports may rely on physical examinations or multiphasic screening that are extremely expensive and cannot readily be used in the epidemiologic study of fairly rare but disabling diseases. Screening techniques have also been criticized on several grounds.[24]

Of immediate concern, such screenings are more likely to identify patients with diseases of moderate progression, which last long enough to be picked up by the screening, than those with rapidly progressive diseases who become ill and die between screenings. So the relatively good treatment results in the number of cases identified by screening is partly a reflection of a bias in the type of cases that screenings identify.

Another concern is that when screening identifies a patient in the preclinical stages of an illness for which there is no effective treatment, survival is counted from that point on. Survival then is bound to be longer than in a patient identified only when his disease becomes clinical. However, what has been added is not years or months of survival; it is years or months of illness.

Finally, it is well known that the cost of community surveys and screening programs is high, and in the opinion of many epidemiologists, the cost-benefit analysis has not been definitely proven to be positive.[25] One way to cut down on cost has been to use key informants; that is, to identify sick individuals through the reports of community leaders or persons who by their occupation are familiar with health problems. This is adequate in small communities where duplications can be easily identified, where the population is relatively stable, and where everybody knows everybody else's business. It is obviously not adequate in large urban areas.[26]

## SOCIAL INDICATORS AND HEALTH STATUS DETERMINATION

Ecologic statistics have also been used to give an indication of a community's health: records of illegitimate births, arrests, quality of housing, income, and so on. But the critics of what has been called the "ecologic fallacy"[27] have been quick to point out that correlating such indices with health status gives information about aggregates of individuals living in areas but does not direct our attention to specific target populations or conditions. In their recent study in Chicago, Levy and Rowitz reported that areas characterized by a high proportion of people under 25, high proportion of blacks, high illegitimacy rates, high delinquency rates, etc. had significantly higher rates of hospitalization for mental disorders but that the known casualties were white and elderly.[28]

It is obvious that none of the classical indices of health status by themselves are satisfactory. New measures, such as Sullivan's combined index, the "Q" index listed by the Indian Health Service, or those of the Northern Ohio Regional Medical Program or Human Population Laboratory in California, are being proposed.[29] It is possible that methodologic issues will be substantially reduced if not eventually solved by continued efforts in these directions.

## VALIDITY OF ASSUMPTIONS IN HEALTH CARE POLICY PLANNING

Beyond the methodologic issues, there are more basic and substantive issues. Presently we are under tremendous pressure to provide health measurements to allow for better program planning and health care delivery. It has become official policy. Is this justified? Should not the validity assumptions on which this policy is based be reevaluated and questioned?

One of the *first* assumptions is that the measurement of illness will give us a measure of the need for professional intervention. Is it so? We ought to know by now that the majority of conditions are mild, often self-limiting, and even tend to disappear *in spite* of treatment when treated. We know that the frequency of spontaneous resolution is one of the major obstacles to the scientific evaluation of our therapeutic efforts. Yet we continue to ignore it in planning. We also ignore the fact that there often is an effective network of care-givers who are much more acceptable to some populations than are health professionals. This is especially true in underdeveloped countries, but it also occurs in some population subgroups in the West.

The *second* assumption is that we can treat the conditions we identify. Yet there are illnesses for which there is very little we can do to prevent or cure. This is true of some psychiatric conditions; it is also true of many degenerative, chronic, and genetic diseases.

There are dangers, we think, in assessing conditions when we do not have the necessary technology to lessen their impact. For one, we unfairly raise the expectations of people with such conditions. Another danger is that caught in the vise of social research, marketing research, political polling, and health research, people are becoming restive about submitting to what seems to be an endless stream of interviews. Although we use random sampling techniques, it seems that some people are more random than others and find themselves approached for interviews over and over again. They rarely get any feedback, and when the novelty of the interview situation wears off, the nonresponse rate creeps up. For those never selected or interviewed, there is a feeling that the entire world seems to know what ought to be wrong with them, but there is no forum to express their disagreement or opinion. And overall, the tremendous suspicions regarding confidentiality of information must be recognized. We are in danger of losing our respondent population, and responsive populations are a natural resource that must be preserved.

The *third* assumption we question is whether or not communities are so different as to require exact and precise measurement of health for adequate planning. To an extent, we are fooling ourselves when we pretend that it is so; when we pretend we know so little. We do know that the poor, the elderly, the illiterate, and the malnourished are at high risk of infectious disease, mental disorders, etc. and go untreated. For example, in Srole's Midtown Manhattan study only one in twenty of all disabled people identified were in treatment at the time of the survey.[30] In Gruenberg's survey of the elderly in Syracuse, New York, four certifiable cases were found in the community for each case in the hospital.[31] So there are ways to derive an estimate of true morbidity from treated rates.

Although there is danger in extrapolating the results found in one community to another one without correction, there is too much of a tendency to ignore former, solidly established findings. If the sociodemographic make-up of a community for which services are planned is by and large comparable to another for which good data has already been gathered, the assessment of needs should (1) take this data in consideration and (2) gather only the data that is missing and do it well. Extrapolations are permissible and accurate enough when one has absorbed and mastered already available information.

Are we not by compulsively gathering data—too often poor data—overfeeding computers and starving our communities by diverting funds better spent in active care? It is a favorite tool of political immobilism to appoint a committee or a commission when a prickly problem arises or will not go away. Could it be that a new strategy of "do nothingness" will be the design and implementation of needless studies—particularly when findings are ignored and funds are not budgeted to implement programs identified as being needed.

We stress that we have not come to definite conclusions regarding the issues raised. We are not "antihealth needs measurement" oriented people. But we think that before we pour our efforts and resources into need assessment, as professionals, we should carefully examine the implications of our actions.

Measurement and careful thinking should not be dichotomized. Although there are funds and pressure from the government to measure, let's arrive at a sober appraisal of the situation before doing so.

Let us not ignore the information we already have, let us not repeat the mistakes of the past. Let us try to carefully and scientifically design studies focusing on defined problems for which we will gather quality information so that the testing of hypotheses about causal associations leads to new knowledge. Let us carry out randomized clinical or preventive trials. The raison d'etre of epidemiology and public health, after all, is to prevent illness, not to measure it over and over again.

## NOTES

1.  Jones, E. *Papers on psychoanalysis* (4th Ed.). Baltimore: Wood Publishers, 1938.

2.  World Health Organization. *The first ten years of the World Health Organization.* Geneva: World Health Organization, 1958.

3.  Callahan, D. The WHO Definition of "health." *The Hastings Center Studies,* 1973, *1*(3), 77–78.

4.  Dubos, R. *Mirage of health: Utopias, progress and biological change.* Garden City, N.Y. Doubleday, 1959, p. 13.

5.  Lewis, A. Health as a social concept. *British Journal of Sociology,* 1953, *4,* 109–124.

6.  Sullivan, D. F. *Conceptual problems in developing an index of health.* (Public Health Service Publication 1000, Series 2, No. 17). Washington, D.C.: U.S. Government Printing Office, 1966, p. 5.

7.  Sigerist, H. E. Socialized medicine. In Me. E. Roemer (Ed.), *On the sociology of medicine.* New York: M. D. Publications, 1960.

8.  Hoyman, J. S. *Our modern concept of health.* Paper presented at the American Public Health Association Annual Meeting, Detroit, Michigan, November 16, 1961.

9.  Wylie, C. M. The definition and measurement of health and disease. *Public Health Reports,* 1970, *85,* 101–104.

10. Romano, J. Basic orientation and education of medical students. *JAMA,* 1950, *143,* 109–112.

11. Dorn, H. F. Methods of measuring incidence and prevalence of disease. *American Journal of Public Health,* 1951, *41,* 271–278.

12. Elinson, J. Methods of socio-medical research. In H. E. Freeman, S. Levine, & L. G. Reeder (Eds.), *Handbook of medical sociology* (2nd Ed.). Englewood Cliffs, N.J.: Prentice-Hall, 1972.

13. Moriyama, I. M. Problems in the measurement of health status. In W. Moore, & E. Sheldon (Eds.), *Indicators of social change.* New York: Russell Sage Foundation, 1968, p. 595.

14. Anonymous. Coroners and suicide. *British Medical Journal,* 1975, *3,* 238–239.

15. Lilienfeld, A. M., Levin, M. L., & Kessler, I. *Cancer in the United States, vital & health statistics.* Cambridge, Massachusetts: Harvard University Press, 1972, (monograph).

16. Jarvis, E. Influence of distance from and nearness to our insane hospital on its use by the people. *American Journal of Insanity,* 1866, *22,* 361.

17. Monteiro, L. A. Expense is no object . . . income and physician visits reconsidered. *Journal of Health and Social Behavior,* 1973, *14,* 99–115.

18. Tooth, G. C. & Brooke, E. M. Trends in the mental hospital population and their effect on planning. *Lancet*, 1961, *1*, 710–713.

19. Gruenberg, E. M. & Turns, D. Epidemiology. In A. M. Freeman, H. I. Kaplan, & B. J. Sadock (Eds.), *Comprehensive Textbook of Psychiatry/II*. Baltimore: Williams & Wilkins, 1975, 398–413.

20. Berkanovic, E. & Reeder, L. G. Ethnic, economic, and social psychological factors in the source of medical care. *Social Problems*, 1973, *21*, 246–259.

21. McKinlay, J. B. Some approaches and problems in the study of the use of services—an overview. *Journal of Health and Social Behavior*, 1972, *13*, 115–152.

22. Newby, L. G. Residual health care needs: Relationship of health status and health services' utilization. Unpublished Ph.D. dissertation. Columbus: The Ohio State University, 1977.

23. National Center for Health Statistics. *Reporting of hospitalization in the health interview survey*. (Public Health Service Publication 1000, Series 1, No. 6). Washingtn, D.C.: U.S. Government Printing Office, 1965.

24. Sackett, D. L. Screening for early detection of disease: To what purpose? *Bulletin of the New York Academy of Medicine*, 1975, *51*, 39–52.

25. LeRiche, W. H. & Milner, J. *Epidemiology as medical ecology*. Edinburgh: Churchill Livingstone, 1971, pp. 81–108.

26. Cooper, B. & Morgan, H. G. *Epidemiological psychiatry*. Springfield, Ill.: Charles C. Thomas, 1973.

27. Robinson, W. S. Ecological correlations and the behavior of individuals. In S. M. Lipset & N. J. Smelser (Eds.), *Sociology: The progress of a decade*. Englewood Cliffs, N.J.: Prentice-Hall, 1961.

28. Levy, L. & Rowitz, L. *The ecology of mental disorders*. New York: Behavioral Publications, 1973.

29. Goldsmith, S. E. The status of health status indicators. *Health Services Reports*, 1972, *87*, 212–220.

30. Srole, L., Langner, T. S., Michael, S. T., & Opler, M. K. *Mental health in the metropolis: The Midtown Manhattan Study* (Vol. I). New York: McGraw-Hill, 1962.

31. Staff of the Mental Health Research Unit. *A mental survey of older people*. Utica, N.Y.: State Hospitals Press, 1960.

# Chapter 7

# STRESSFUL LIFE EVENTS AND ILLNESS

## Implications for Need Assessment

*Barbara S. Dohrenwend*

A straightforward approach to need assessment is to attempt to identify people in a community who are currently suffering from physical and psychological disorders and disabilities. Another appealing possibility is to identify those who may be at risk of developing disorders and disabilities. To determine how we might best assess this risk, let us consider the general etiologic model that is becoming accepted for a wide range of serious somatic disorders (e.g., heart disease) as well as psychological disorders (e.g., schizophrenia). This model suggests that environmental stressors act to induce disorders in individuals who are particularly vulnerable to them because of genetic factors or predispositions developed early in life. Vulnerability to disorder, thus established, is either immutable, if genetically determined, or difficult to change, if based on early experience. Therefore, the best hope of preventing many serious health problems seems to be offered by interventions aimed at stressors in the contemporary environment. Among environmental stressors, social stressors appear to be the largest and the least disorder-specific type.

Several reasons suggest that social stressors can usefully be identified by focusing on stressful life events such as a death in the family, a divorce, a job loss, or a change of residence. One reason is that stressful life events apparently have a wide range of effects, as indicated by case-control studies linking them to, among other things, heart disease, fractures, childhood leukemia, schizophrenia, depression, and suicide.[1-7] Another set of reasons is based on the prevalence of psychological disorders in community populations. Despite arguments to the contrary, epidemiologic studies provide no evidence that the overall rate of psychological disorders has increased over time.[8-10] This apparent stability suggests that aspects of the social environment associated with psychological disorders are part of the human condition rather than some perverse invention of twentieth century man. Moreover, since psychological disorders are, at least when broadly defined, not uncommon in the general population, the social conditions to which they are related must be pervasive rather than rare. Stressful life events are indeed a part of the human condition, and they are pervasive.

## MEASUREMENT OF THE MAGNITUDE OF STRESSFUL LIFE EVENTS

Assuming, then, that we want to identify individuals or groups in the community who are at risk of illness because they are exposed to stressful life events, how should we do it? The difficulty we face is suggested by considering some of the strongest evidence for the proposition that stressful experiences can cause physical and psychological disorders and disabilities. Part of this evidence comes from the laboratory. There, a typical procedure is to expose healthy animals to some aversive stimulus, under controlled conditions, and observe their responses. Under suitable combinations of environmental conditions they can be made, among other things, to become helpless—in the sense of giving up attempts to avoid punishment,[11] to develop stomach ulcers, or even to die.[12]

Another source of strong evidence of the effects of a stressful environment is war, appropriately described by Grinker and Spiegel[13] as "a laboratory which manufactures psychological dysfunction." Analysis has shown that combat exhaustion regularly occurred in previously normal soldiers when about 65 percent of their companions had been killed, wounded, or had otherwise become casualties.[14]

The causal inferences to be drawn are clear because, among other things, the subjects were exposed, in the laboratory, to a standard aversive stimulus, or, in battle, to a similar life-threatening situation. We do not question that these stimuli and situations are stressful nor, within broad limits, that the magnitude of their stressfulness is similar for all who are exposed to them.

In contrast, the normal civilian experiences that we label stressful life events are not the same from person to person. One person gets divorced, another loses his job, and a third changes his residence. This specificity is, I think, one reason why the concept of stressful life events is so appealing. Like the case study method, it recognizes qualitative differences in individual lives. At the same time, this characteristic creates one of the most serious methodologic problems in studies of stressful life events, the challenge to develop measures that will permit generalizations about normal life stress that are as unequivocal as those based on contrived laboratory studies or on the horrors of war and other extreme situations. How, then, do we decide whether a relative's death is more stressful than getting divorced, or how these events compare with losing one's job or changing one's residence?

Many readers are probably aware of the attractive solution to this problem offered by Holmes and Rahe in their Social Readjustment Ratings. To secure these ratings they asked 394 judges to rate the amount of readjustment entailed in each of 42 life events relative to marriage, which was designated as the modulus event. Holmes in particular has argued, on the basis of correlations on the order of 0.9 between the mean ratings by judges of contrasting social statuses, that there is a high level of consensus about the magnitudes of these life events.

Having developed their scoring system, Holmes and his colleagues asked subjects in subsequent studies which of the 43 life events they had recently experienced and assigned each subject a life change score by summing the readjustment scores of all reported events. Holmes and Masuda concluded, "The greater the magnitude of life change . . . the greater the probability that the life change would be associated with disease onset, and the greater the probability that the population at risk would experience disease."[5]

We apparently have, then, a ready procedure for determining who is at risk of illness in terms of exposure to stressful life events. The findings of Holmes and his colleagues indicate that we should not take the occurrence of any life event, regardless of its magnitude, as indicative of risk. Instead, events at the upper end of the Social Readjustment Rating Scale, such as a death in the family, or serious marital difficulties, are the ones that seem to indicate the need for intervention.

### EXAMPLES OF INTERVENTION PROGRAMS BASED ON THE OCCURRENCE OF STRESSFUL LIFE EVENTS

Intervention programs based on this conception of need have been rare. We can, however, learn a great deal from the few that have been designed and implemented.

One of these programs was developed in the context of the Vietnam war. Originally named Operation Egress Recap and later Operation Homecoming, this program was designed by military psychiatrists to prevent the development of severe psychological disorders among returning American prisoners of war. Every ex-prisoner was to spend a few days in an overseas military hospital before returning to the states, with the rationale, as reported in the *New York Times*, that, "By delaying family reunions and other emotional encounters—or even any requirement for the simplest acts of decision-making—it is hoped to provide the isolation needed for effective medical and psychological treatment."[15] Given the context of this program there were, of course, political protests.[16,17] In addition, however, the protests against delayed reunions by some of the men and their families suggest that the military psychiatrists' definition of need did not entirely coincide with the target population's definition of want.[17] As a consequence at least in part of this resistance, this program was never fully implemented. In the weeks and months immediately after their return, however, suicides by several exprisoners tragically suggested that there may have been an unmet need for help.

Before deciding what we can learn from this experience, let us look at the somewhat different results of an experimental program that provided crisis intervention for families in which there had been a sudden death.[18] In this controlled experiment, one group of families who experienced a sudden death received crisis intervention, while the remaining families experiencing a sudden death in the same time period received no intervention. When the experimental and control families were compared six months after the death, the investigators found that crisis intervention "did not . . . lower the incidence of medical and psychiatric illness or of disturbed social functioning in bereaved families."[19] At the same time, the existence of need was suggested by the observation that six months after the death[19]

> Family members in both bereaved groups showed poorer functioning in several areas than non-bereaved families—both groups of bereaved families had significantly greater acting out . . ., greater depression . . ., and greater problems in family, intrapersonal, interpersonal, and social functioning . . .

In contrast to Operation Homecoming, there apparently was no resistance by any of the bereaved families. Instead, evaluation of this experimental program revealed the ineffectiveness of the services provided.

So far we have assumed that there is only one model—that stressful life events contribute to the development of a wide variety of disorders and disabilities, many of them serious. At this point, it will be useful to consider an alternative for the light it throws on another problem to be solved if assessment of needs is to be based on stressful life events.

This alternate model, developed in the context of psychiatric epidemiology, focuses on the problem of explaining reports that the prevalence of psychological disorder in some communities, and in some groups within communities, is well over 50 percent. These high rates are explained in terms of a process whereby stressful life events induce psychological symptoms that are transient but, while they last, indistinguishable from symptoms of chronic and sometimes serious psychopathology.[20,21] The importance of this model for our purposes is what it implies about the need for intervention. In contrast to the previous model, it suggests that people recently exposed to stressful life events should be identified not so that they can be helped, but so that they will not mistakenly be labeled as mentally ill and provided with unnecessary treatment. The importance of guarding against treating potentially transient stress reactions as if they indicated psychopathology is supported by observations during World Wars I and II that men receiving traditional psychotherapy for psychological manifestations of combat exhaustion often developed chronic war neuroses, while those treated as if their reactions were transient generally did not develop a permanent disability.[22]

This experience in two World Wars, together with the problems revealed by Operation Homecoming and the experimental intervention program for bereaved families, are, I think, sufficient to call into question the definition of need simply in terms of the occurrence of highly stressful life events that apparently increase the risk of illness. We have seen that this definition can generate resistance among those designated as in need, does not seem to provide a basis for designing effective interventions, and holds the potential of dictating interventions when they may be harmful rather than helpful. Let us go back, then, to the work of Holmes and his colleagues and see if we can locate the source of these problems and develop a solution.

## AN ALTERNATIVE PROCEDURE FOR ASSESSING THE STRESSFULNESS OF LIFE EVENTS

Holmes' and Rahe's work was a major methodologic breakthrough in the study of stressful life events. It has, however, been the target of a number of well-taken criticisms. One issue that has received a great deal of attention concerns the way in which Holmes and his colleagues conceptualized the stressfulness of an event. While they argued that the stressfulness of a life event inheres in the amount of change entailed,[4,23] some critics have countered that it derives primarily from an event's undesirability.[24,25] In fact, the two characteristics are highly correlated, with undesirable life events generally judged as involving more change than desirable events.[26,27] Furthermore, there is evidence that the power of change measures to predict the onset of disorders and disabilities is largely limited to undesirable events.[25,26] It might be useful, therefore, to combine undesirability ratings with change ratings instead of using only one to measure stressfulness. This procedure would not, however, solve the problems revealed by the intervention programs that we reviewed, since they were all based on undesirable events that entailed major readjustment.

Another criticism that may be more pertinent to the problems with which we are concerned questions the assumption that the event scores derived from ratings made by 394 judges are equally accurate for all individuals and groups. The alternate position, that seems to have gained wide acceptance, is that the magnitude of an event depends crucially on the meaning of the event to the person who experiences it.[28] A quantitative procedure based on this premise is Rahe's Subjective Life Change Unit Method, whereby a subject is asked to rate each of his recent life events on a scale from zero to one hundred to indicate "the amount of adjustment (he) needed to handle the event."[29]

This subjective approach, whether quantitative or not, seems to be eminently unsuitable for need assessment because the meaning of these measures is ambiguous and may be irrelevant. Consider, for example, the finding that patients with recent heart attacks gave higher ratings than nonpatient controls to events that preceded the heart attacks.[30] The most plausible interpretation is that the cardiac patients retrospectively exaggerated the stressfulness of their life events as a means of explaining their heart attacks. Another possibility is to interpret the relatively high patient ratings as reflections of a personality trait associated with proneness to heart attack. Another is to assume that the events experienced by cardiac patients actually were objectively greater in magnitude; but even if we were to make this somewhat implausible assumption, the patients' ratings would not indicate anything about the greater magnitude of their life events which could be used to reduce heart attack incidence. None of these interpretations suggests, then, that subjective ratings provide a measure of objective environmental stressors on which program planners could base a determination of needs for preventive intervention.

Even though we reject the usefulness of subjective ratings of recently experienced life events for need assessment and program planning, we should not overlook the major argument in their favor, which is that they provide better predictions of illness than Holmes' and Rahe's standard of life event ratings. This superior accuracy of prediction is based, it is argued, on a more accurate estimate of the stressfulness of particular life events as they are actually experienced.

Criticism of Holmes' and Rahe's ratings has been made by George Brown from another perspective leading him to propose a different solution, based on objective measures, for improving the estimate of risk. He has pointed out that Holmes and Rahe provide minimal and often highly ambiguous information about the life events they study:

> The descriptions used to rate degree of readjustment made necessary by the event are brief. A person simply begins or stops work; we do not know whether the change is forced or voluntary, whether due to the birth of a baby, a husband's antagonism, or winning money in the lottery, whether it means losing important ties or the need to make new ones, or whether the change is the first or had occurred many times before.[2]

Brown has argued that to obtain a more accurate determination of what effect a life event is likely to have, we need to describe not only the event itself but also the objective circumstances in which it occurred, since these circumstances can be expected to mediate the impact of the event on the individual. To this end he has proposed a procedure for rating the objective circumstances surrounding a life event.

In the first step of Brown's procedure, the subject is encouraged by an interviewer to talk freely about a recent life event and its circumstances. The interviewer does not ask preset questions but guides the subject to provide information in 30 categories, which cover " . . . three main areas: (1) prior experience and preparation; (2) immediate reactions; and (3) the consequences and implications of the event."[3] To obtain ratings that are not influenced by the subject's feelings about the event, his descriptions of his reactions are edited from the interview record, leaving only descriptions of the event and its objective circumstances. Finally, a team of specially trained researchers make two ratings of "contextual threat," one for short-term and one for long-term threat, on the basis of hearing the edited interview. These ratings are made on a four point scale of "marked," "moderate," "some," or "little or no" threat. The raters are guided by examples that illustrate the four ratings and by conventions which usually apply to certain events. The final ratings are determined by the agreement reached among the raters after any differences are resolved by discussion.

This procedure does deal with the objective circumstances of an event. The potential user is frustrated, however, by the extent to which it involves mystification of measurement. The uninitiated do not know with any precision what data is presented by the interviewer to the raters, or even whether it is comparable from one case to the next. Nor do the uninitiated have any way of understanding how the raters synthesize the complex of circumstances into the ultimate ratings of short-term and long-term contextual threat.

The advantage of these ratings, like subjects' own ratings of the magnitudes of their life events, is that prediction of the effects of the events is improved when they are used. However, these synthetic ratings do not indicate which aspects of life event contexts are most likely to increase or, equally important, decrease the risk of developing disorders and disabilities.

It seems to me that George Brown has asked the right question but come up with the wrong answer. We do need to know more about the circumstances that might cushion or aggravate the impact of an event on an individual, but we need to measure specific circumstances so that we can develop explicit principles on which to base these estimates of risk. I propose that we be guided in specifying these circumstances by some very strong leads in the general research literature on stress. Let me describe four leads that I think are promising.

In his criticism of the vagueness of Holmes' and Rahe's descriptions of life events, Brown noted, among other things, that " . . . we do not know . . . whether the change is the first or had occurred many times before."[2] This omission is important because defining the stressfulness of an event by the amount of change it entails implies that an event that "had occurred many times before" would be less stressful than one experienced for the first time. This implication may not hold for all events, regardless of their undesirability, that is, the repetition of undesirable events may sometimes increase rather than reduce their stressfulness. We do not know how many times a particular event must be experienced before habituation occurs. The general proposition that habituation reduces stress has, however, been solidly established in extensive research on the psychology of learning.

Earlier, it was noted that some of the strongest evidence that stressful experiences can cause disorders and disabilities comes from observations of the effects of battle on soldiers. The specific observation was cited that combat exhaustion regularly occurred in previously normal soldiers when about 65 percent of their companions had been killed, wounded, or had otherwise become casualties.[14] Further evidence of the protective effect of social bonds is found in a study which showed that, among women who experienced stressful life events before or during their pregnancies, those with more satisfactory marital and other social relations were less likely than those with less satisfactory relations to suffer complications in their pregnancies.[31] That effects analogous to those observed in humans have been demonstrated in laboratory studies of animals suggests that social bonds provide a fundamental buffer against the impact of stressful situations.[32] The results of all of these studies, in and out of the laboratory, strongly imply that the effects of a stressful life event cannot be predicted without information about the social context in which it is experienced.[32] Clearly, then, we can improve our estimates of risk taking this factor into account.

Two other conditions that may mediate the impact of life events are suggested by recent reviews of laboratory studies of stress.[33,34] The first is anticipation of a noxious stimulus. When a subject is able to anticipate such a stimulus, either because a warning is provided or because of the regular timing of the stimulus, effects of the stimulus are mitigated. To illustrate, one study showed that a fixed-interval noise produced less deterioration in performance on a subsequent proofreading task than did a random noise and that, in addition, this difference in regularity had a far greater impact on subsequent performance than the loudness of the noise.[35]

Another generally consistent experimental finding is that when a subject controls the administration of a noxious stimulus, its effects are ameliorated. Thus, for example, when subjects were told that they could turn off a loud, random noice if it became unbearable, they performed better at a subsequent proofreading task than when they had no control over the noxious stimulus.[35]

Given the highly artificial settings of experimental studies such as these and, of ethical necessity, the rather trivial nature of the stressful experiences imposed, the question arises as to whether these findings can be generalized to life situations. Evidence to answer this question is provided by an extensive series of clinical cases collected by Schmale and his colleagues,[36] who concluded that people who feel helpless to anticipate and control their world are particularly likely to suffer serious illness or even death when stressful events impinge on them. Experimental and clinical findings both suggest, then, that differences in the extent to which stressful life events are anticipated or their onset controlled may explain some of the variability in their impact.

## EXPERIENCE WITH SYSTEMATIC MEASURES OF ANTICIPATION AND CONTROL OF LIFE EVENTS

The experimental and clinical literature on stress, as well as studies of extreme situations, imply that reactions to a stressful life event cannot be understood without taking into account contextual factors such as amount of previous experience with the event and social support available, and the degree of anticipation and control of the occurrence of the event. The implication is that we should measure these factors if we want to assess needs that are generated by stressful life events. In a study in New York City, we are working with the contextual factors of anticipation and control of the occurrence of life events. Let me describe some measurement problems that we have encountered, and some partial solutions that we have developed to illustrate the methodologic tangle that must be undone in order to examine the circumstances surrounding stressful life events.

We encountered the first kink when we set out to create a standardized interview to measure, among other things, the extent of respondents' anticipation and control of their life events. We found, as you would expect, that questions about anticipation and control could be standardized in that all respondents could be asked the same question about a given event. However, it soon became obvious that if any one question was asked about all events, it would, in many instances, sound either absurd or threatening. For example, we could ask a respondent whether it was entirely his decision to start a new business, but could not reasonably ask the same question if his business had failed. Instead, the only sensible question seemed to be whether he could have done something to prevent the failure. After some reworking, we found that two questions concerning anticipation and three concerning control were sufficient to provide forms that were neither absurd nor threatening in relation to any of the 102 events on our list.[37]

The use of different questions for different kinds of events creates a problem, however. This procedure deviates from the conventional concept of standardization of measurement because it may confound differences in questions with differences in responses. Suppose, for example, that we find that respondents generally report more control over starting new businesses than over business failures. This difference could be due to the nature of the two events or to the different questions we asked about them. In practice, the overlapping arrays of life events that respondents report in actual interviews provide some leverage for dealing with this issue insofar as it affects the interpretation of individual and group differences.[37] At the very least, however, this necessary compromise with standardization complicates the analysis of data on the anticipation and control of the occurrence of life events. Nevertheless, this explicit and systematic variation in questions seems preferable to allowing questions to vary in unknown ways as a function of the inventiveness of individual interviewers; the latter procedure hides the methodologic problem rather than solving it.

Another problem presented by these contextual measures of the anticipation and control of the occurrences of life events is that they cannot be assumed *a priori* to measure objective circumstances rather than subjective predispositions. Thus, for example, when we ask a respondent whether he could have prevented the failure of his business, is his negative answer an expression of his predisposition to blame others rather than himself, or is it an objective assessment of conditions that caused his business to fail? Analyses of data that we have collected in our study provide both reassurance and a caution on this question. They indicate that there was a large measure of objectivity in the reports that respondents gave about control of the onset of their life events. That is, insofar as we were able to explain variations in reported levels of control, these explanations involved objective situational variables, such as the respondent's role in the event, rather than personal characteristics of the respondents giving the reports. In contrast, we found that reports of anticipation of stressful life events were in part determined by a characteristic of the reporter. Specifically, reported levels of anticipation varied with ethnicity; Puerto Ricans reporting lower levels of certainty prior to the occurrence of their life events than non-Puerto Rican blacks and whites.[37]

The point that I want to emphasize is that, given systematic measurement of explicit circumstances, we can develop general principles about the variation in these circumstances and apply them to estimates of risk arising from stressful life events. Thus, for example, we can take this ethnic difference in tendency to anticipate stressful life events into account if we are concerned about the effects of these events on an ethnically heterogeneous population.

## THE IMPLICATIONS OF FACTORS THAT MEDIATE THE IMPACT OF STRESSFUL LIFE EVENTS FOR NEEDS ASSESSMENT

I would like to return now to the problems that we identified in programs and policies based on the assumption that highly stressful life events create needs for health and human services regardless of the circumstances of the events. Let us consider how information about the specific circumstances of life events might help to solve these problems.

One problem is to avoid directing interventions at individuals whose responses to a stressful life event are transient and, conversely, to focus on individuals who are not likely to recover spontaneously. Evidence suggests that knowledge of the circumstances of an event could help to provide this focus. Thus, for example, in the experiment with bereaved families the investigators found that the presence, six months after the death, of physical and mental illness in the family or of serious family disruption was correlated with, among other things, the death being extremely sudden, and with lack of an effective network of social support outside the family.[18] Selective intervention in families thus identified would presumably help to reduce the risk of inappropriate labeling and treatment of transient responses to a death in the family.

In Operation Homecoming the proffered services were actively rejected by some of the exprisoners and their families. On the other hand, some of the families were prepared to cooperate with the program.[15] If the need for help had been defined in terms of the circumstances to which particular exprisoners were returning as well as the mere fact of the return from imprisonment in Vietnam, it might have been possible to distinguish those who wanted help from those who construed the program as an intrusion. Moreover, if the need for intervention had been specified more precisely, it would not have been as easy as it was to accuse the military psychiatrists of designing a program based on political rather than medical considerations.

A better understanding of the circumstances of life events that create a need for help should also provide a basis for designing more effective intervention. In Operation Homecoming, the plan apparently was to offer psychotherapy, which seems to have been a mistake, given the experiences in two World Wars that we noted previously. In contrast, the investigators who conducted the experiment with bereaved families explicitly did not offer traditional psychotherapy. Their approach, instead, was to offer whatever services seemed to be needed with, apparently, no detailed preconception about what those services might be. The ineffectiveness of this approach suggests that we need to develop some clear preconceptions about services to be offered. Specifically, these services might be designed to counteract the effects of the circumstances surrounding an event that would otherwise be expected to amplify the impact of the event.

## CONCLUSION

I think it has become apparent that the argument for choosing stressful life events as a basis for assessing needs is not that they can be measured with ready procedures that are easy to use, but that they imply a commitment to the goal of reducing the incidence of stress-induced illness in the community we serve. Many of us have been hoping, particularly since the publication by Holmes and Rahe in 1967 of the results of their Social Readjustment Rating Questionnaire, that both arguments could be made at the same time, that a readily administered and easily scored checklist of life events would indicate what is required to prevent the onset of stress induced illness. From the start, however, this hope has lacked substance. The prediction that illness will probably follow if an individual is exposed to a sufficient quantity of life stress encourages resignation rather than the prescription of preventive measures.

We got caught in this trap, I think, because we were so distracted by the complex methodologic problems inherent in studying life events that we lost contact with the larger body of stress theory and research. If we had been investigating stress in the laboratory, we would not have predicted, for example, that the higher the voltage used to shock an animal, the greater the probability of his becoming helpless regardless of the conditions under which the shocks were delivered. Surely if it is necessary to specify these contextual conditions to predict the effect of electric shock on a laboratory animal, it is just as necessary to specify the circumstances that cushion or amplify the impact of life events in order to understand their effects. Moreover, I suggest that this necessity shows us the way out of the trap in which we have been floundering, for the circumstances that amplify or cushion the impact of stressful life events provide a foundation on which we can build programs of need assessment and related services designed to reduce the incidence of stress-induced illness in the communities we serve. On the cornerstone of this foundation is written: Though life stress is inevitable, stress-induced illness is not.

## NOTES

1. Brown, G. W. Meaning, measurement, and stress of life events. In B. S. Dohrenwend & B. P. Dohrenwend (Eds.), *Stressful life events.* New York: Wiley, 1974, pp. 217–244.

2. *Ibid.,* p. 221.

3. *Ibid.,* p. 229.

4. Holmes, T. H., & Masuda, M. Life change and illness susceptibility. In B. S. Dohrenwend & B. P. Dohrenwend (Eds.), *Stressful life events.* New York: Wiley, 1974, pp. 45–72.

5. *Ibid.,* p. 68.

6. Hudgens, R. W. Personal catastrophe and depression: A consideration of the subject with respect to medically ill adolescents, and a requiem for retrospective life-event studies. In B. S. Dohrenwend & B. P. Dohrenwend (Eds.), *Stressful life events.* New York: Wiley, 1974, pp. 119–134.

7. Paykel, E. S. Life stress and psychiatric disorder: Applications of the clinical approach. In B. S. Dohrenwend & B. P. Dohrenwend (Eds.), *Stressful life events.* New York: Wiley, 1974, pp. 135–150.

8. Dohrenwend, B. P., & Dohrenwend, B. S. Social and cultural influences on psychopathology. *Annual Review of Psychology,* 1974, *25,* 417–452.

9. Dohrenwend, B. P., & Dohrenwend, B. S. Sex differences and psychiatric disorders. *American Journal of Sociology,* 1976, *81,* 1447–1454.

10. Schwab, J. J., & Schwab, R. B. The epidemiology of mental illness. In G. Usdin (Ed.), *Psychiatry, education, and image.* New York: Academic Press, 1973, pp. 58–83.

11.  Seligman, M. E. P. *Helplessness: On depression, development and death.* San Francisco: Freeman, 1975.

12.  Selye, H. *The stress of life.* New York: McGraw-Hill, 1956.

13.  Grinker, R. R., & Spiegel, J. P. *Men under stress.* New York: McGraw-Hill, 1963, p. 8.

14.  Swank, R. L. Combat exhaustion. *Journal of Nervous and Mental Disease,* 1949, *109,* 475–508.

15.  Holles, E. R. U.S. planned more gradual homecoming for P.O.W. *New York Times,* September 30, 1972, p. 10.

16.  Hersh, S. M. Freed pilots begin tests and are visited by families. *New York Times,* September 30, 1972, p. 10.

17.  Roberts, S. V. War foes assail plans on P.O.W.'s *New York Times,* December 10, 1972, p. 8.

18.  Polak, P. R., Egan, D., Vandenbergh, R., & Williams, W. V. Prevention in mental health: A controlled study. *American Journal of Psychiatry,* 1975, *132,* 146–149.

19.  *Ibid.,* p. 147.

20.  Dohrenwend, B. S. Social status and stressful life events. *Journal of Personality and Social Psychology,* 1973, *28,* 225–235.

21.  Myers, J. K., Lindenthal, J. J., & Pepper, M. P. Social class, life events, and psychiatric symptoms: A longitudinal study. In B. S. Dohrenwend & B. P. Dohrenwend (Eds.), *Stressful life events.* New York: Wiley, 1974, pp. 191–205.

22.  Glass, A. J. Psychotherapy in the combat zone. In *Symposium on stress.* Washington, D.C.: Army Medical Service Graduate School, 1953, pp. 284–294.

23.  Holmes, T. H., & Rahe, R. H. The social readjustment rating scale. *Journal of Psychosomatic Research,* 1967, *11,* 213–218.

24.  Gersten, J. G., Langner, T. S., Eisenberg, J. G., & Orzek, L. Child behavior and life events: Undesirable change or change per se? In B. S. Dohrenwend & B. P. Dohrenwend (Eds.), *Stressful life events.* New York: Wiley, 1974, pp. 159–170.

25.  Vinokur, A., & Selzer, M. L. Desirable versus undesirable life events; their relationship to stress and mental distress. *Journal of Personality and Social Psychology,* 1975, *32,* 329–337.

26. Dohrenwend, B. S. Life events as stressors: A methodological inquiry. *Journal of Health and Social Behavior*, 1973, *14*, 167–175.

27. Hough, R. L., Fairbank, D. T., & Garcia, A. M. Problems in the ratio measurement of life stress. *Journal of Health and Social Behavior*, 1976, *17*, 70–82.

28. Hinkle, L. E., Jr. The effect of exposure to culture change, social change, and changes in interpersonal relationships on health. In B. S. Dohrenwend & B. P. Dohrenwend (Eds.), *Stressful life events*. New York: Wiley, 1974, pp. 9–44.

29. Rahe, R. H. The pathway between subjects' recent life changes and their near-future illness reports: Representative results and methodological issues. In B. S. Dohrenwend & B. P. Dohrenwend (Eds.), *Stressful life events*. New York: Wiley, 1974, pp. 76–77.

30. Theorell, T. Life events before and after the onset of premature myocardial infarction. In B. S. Dohrenwend & B. P. Dohrenwend (Eds.), *Stressful life events*. New York: Wiley, 1974, pp. 101–117.

31. Nuckolls, K. B., Cassel, J., & Kaplan, B. H. Psychosocial assets, life crisis and the prognosis of pregnancy. *American Journal of Epidemiology*, 1972, *95*, 431–441.

32. Cassel, J. Social science in epidemiology: Psychosocial processes and "stress" theoretical formulation. In E. L. Struening & M. Guttentag (Eds.), *Handbook of evaluation research* (Vol. 1). Beverly Hills, Ca.: Sage Publications, 1975, pp. 537–549.

33. Averill, J. R. Personal control over aversive stimuli and its relationship to stress. *Psychological Bulletin*, 1973, *80*, 286–202.

34. Lefcourt, H. M. The function of the illusions of control and freedom. *American Psychologist*, 1973, *28*, 417–425.

35. Glass, D. C., Singer, J. E., & Friedman, L. N. Psychic cost of adaptation to an environmental stressor. *Journal of Personality and Social Psychology*, 1969, *12*, 200–210.

36. Schmale, A. H. Giving up as a final common pathway to changes in health. *Advances in Psychosomatic Medicine*, 1972, *8*, 20–40.

37. Dohrenwend, B. S. Anticipation and control of stressful life events. In J. S. Strauss, H. M. Babigian, & M. Roff (Eds.), *The origins and course of psychopathology*. New York: Plenum Press, 1977.

# Part III

# METHODOLOGICAL ASPECTS OF NEED ASSESSMENT

## INTRODUCTION

A wide variety of techniques have been borrowed from the behavioral and social sciences for need assessment purposes. Four strategies that are among the more widely used are presented and discussed in this section: (1) social indicators, (2) client utilization, (3) field surveys, and (4) nominal group technique. Descriptions of each approach, as well as its advantages and disadvantages, are provided in four of the chapters. In addition, the specific application and results of one technique are presented in the chapter by Zautra, Kochanowicz, and Goodhart.

After discussing several conceptualizations of need, Bloom defines social indicators as measures of social problems (or their absence) and, in their aggregate, measures that form an indication of the quality of life of communities. Bloom points out that the different sets of social indicators that have been used to monitor communities reflect the diversity of conceptualizations of need. These indicators are usually chosen by inductive rather than deductive procedures. They can be used for improving descriptive reporting, analytical studies of social change, and future actuarial predictions. However, they do lack a theoretical base and suffer from vagueness.

Client analysis, as presented by Scheff, involves a conceptual base and method for determining health planning needs and the mechanisms through which services are delivered. To provide background for the discussion of client analysis, Scheff identifies a number of concepts that have historically dominated health planning. Six categories of social planning are also discussed as well as their requirements. The necessary steps that constitute client analysis are identified by Scheff as well as the utility of the approach for identifying needs and planning health services.

While field survey methods, as Warheit and Bell point out, have a number of advantages over other need assessment techniques, they have been criticized at both theoretical and methodologic levels. These criticisms are directly addressed by the authors, and the distinct advantages of the field survey approach are identified. The use of field surveys in conjunction with other approaches—such as key informants, rates-under-treatment, and social indicators—are also discussed. Zautra, Kochanowicz, and Goodhart describe the results of their survey, which was designed to study the quality of life in a community, and identify the potential utility of this approach as an aid in the planning of community mental health services.

The nominal group approach, described by Delbecq, is a useful technique for gathering information in small groups that can be used in understanding the qualitative dimensions of client needs. Such information can be used to identify needs and plan health and human services. This technique involves a highly structured sequence of steps which allows participation by all group members, minimizes status differences among them, minimizes group domination by highly aggressive or verbal individuals, and often produces more data and creative ideas than are produced in unstructured discussion groups.

The common thread which ties these chapters together is a concern for method validity, method reliability, and the utility of the resulting data. Continuing attention to these issues, as demonstrated by the authors in this as well as the preceding and following sections, will contribute to the integration of a presently diverse field.

*Chapter 8*

# THE USE OF SOCIAL INDICATORS IN THE ESTIMATION OF HEALTH NEEDS*

## Bernard L. Bloom

The term *need* is used in two very different ways. First, the term is used synonymously with the term *demand* or *want,* that is, need as assessed by the subject: "I need a doctor," or "My community needs more recreational facilities for 'teen-agers.'" Used in this way, needs may sometimes be converted into action. A person may make an appointment with a physician or may write a letter or form a committee with the purpose of increasing recreational opportunities. The term *need* is used in a second sense to represent expert outside judgment about someone else: "John needs to improve his grades in mathematics if he ever hopes to get into college," or "Based on our studies of medical care, this community needs approximately 100 additional hospital beds." In this sense, the assessment of need is made by the professional rather than the client.

*This chapter is a revision of a presentation delivered at the Louisville National Conference on Need Assessment in Health and Human Services, Louisville, Kentucky, March, 1976. This revision draws on material previously published in *Community mental health: A general introduction.* Monterey, Ca.: Brooks Cole, 1977 and copyrighted by Brooks Cole. Permission to use this material is gratefully acknowledged.

These two strategies of need assessment often yield inconsistent results and there can be an inherent conflict between the client system and the service provider system as to where the primary locus of need assessment should be found. The professional might argue, "I know what you need". The client might argue, "I know what I want. If you won't give it to me, I'll find someone who will".

The professional expert has long had the greater power in need assessment. It is only relatively recently that mental health professionals have sought to discover what their clients or potential clients want. The private practice model is one, after all, in which a service is offered, and as long as the practitioner develops an adequate income, there is little interest in identifying unmet needs. Mental health clinics and community mental health centers developed within this entrepreneurial heritage. With few exceptions, these agencies saw themselves as the primary source of wisdom regarding community mental health related needs. As a result, the most common sequence in developing staffing patterns was to decide that this center with this budget needed so many professional, support, and administrative staff, and then only later, if at all, to attempt to identify community needs to which they might be responsive.

There are serious problems with both definitions. People sometimes do not know what they need. A sense of helplessness or an inability to pay for care can lead to low expression of need. Needs are transient, and felt needs are constantly being manipulated. Experts are people too and can have faulty or outdated information. Fashion can dictate need assessments by experts; and experts have their own biases and motives. Finally, there may be considerable disagreement among experts as to what a particular community or person needs in the service of resolving a particular problem.

There are further complexities defining and assessing needs. There are recognized versus unrecognized needs; met versus unmet needs; private versus public needs; short-term versus long-term needs; and often conflicting needs within a person or within an organization. Need assessment is thus complex, highly political, often irrational and conflictual, and extremely value laden. The hope of the social indicators movement is to detach need assessment from these problems by stepping back and developing a statistical overview of a specific population, community, or society.

## History of Social Indicators

The systematic and regular collection of community information has a long tradition. The United States census has occurred every decade for nearly 200 years and now includes a large number of questions about social conditions. Over one hundred years ago, Herbert Spencer[2] called for the collection and analysis of data on such variables as religion, culture, styles of life, and use of leisure time, suggesting that

> These facts, given with as much brevity as consists with clearness and accuracy, should be so grouped and arranged that they may be comprehended in their ensemble, and contemplated as mutually dependent parts of one great whole. The aim should be so to present them that men may readily trace the consensus subsisting among them with the view of learning what social phenomena coexist with what others.

While Spencer's interest was primarily theoretical, interest in applying social variable analysis began in the late 1920s under the auspices of the federal government. These studies, it was then hoped, might help identify (1) sources of social stress and (2) strategies for reducing them. Interrupted by the depression and the Second World War, interest in the analysis of social variables reappeared after the war, first at the level of the United Nations and subsequently within the United States.

The phrase, social indicators, is generally attributed to Bauer who in 1966 edited a book by that title.[3] Since then the term has gained wide usage. Indeed, a 1972 annotated social indicators bibliography contained more than 1,000 items of which more than half were published since 1970.[4] Sheldon and Parke[5] have suggested that such terms as social indicators or social reporting emerged from an awareness of rapid social change, from a sense of emerging problems with origins deep in the social structure, and from . . . a commitment to the idea that the benefits and costs of domestic social programs are subject to measurement and to the belief that each newly perceived, albeit ancient, inadequacy in the society should, and would, call forth a corrective response from a federal government whose efficacy would be assisted by social measurement, planning and new management analytical techniques.

The most widely known definition is found in a federal publication entitled *Toward a Social Report:*[6]

(a social indicator) . . . a statistic . . . which facilitates concise, comprehensive and balanced judgments about the condition of major aspects of a society. It is in all cases a direct measure of welfare and is subject to the interpretation that, if it changes in the "right" direction, while other things remain equal, things have gotten better, or people are "better off."

The social indicator is thus a measure of social problems (or their absence) and, in the aggregate, an indication of the quality of life. By taking such measures over time, it should be clear whether social problems in a community are getting better or worse. Presumably, a problem could be identified as being so severe that there would be a call to action, and subsequent measurements of the problem could serve to evaluate the effectiveness of the action program. Thus, social indicators, if properly chosen, can serve to evaluate the effectiveness of the action program. Thus, social indicators, if properly chosen, can serve the same function at the community level as such individual indicators as body temperature or I.Q. In a recent review of the literature, Oborn[7] suggests that

the two most important uses of social indicators stressed by writers at all levels are: (1) as guides in decision-making or policy making; and (2) as aids in evaluation of current programs.

## SELECTION OF SOCIAL INDICATORS

The social indicators movement is an effort to develop an assessment procedure parallel and complimentary to the highly successful economic indicators or economic index. Economic theory is relatively well developed and the complex consequences of, for example, increasing unemployment or decreasing wholesale prices are fairly well understood. Accordingly, the use of an economic indicator such as unemployment rate is well justified. Kahn[8] has proposed that the development of social indicators could

> to some degree, correct the incomplete or inaccurate picture of society derived from economic indicators alone and begin to remedy a tendency to underinvest in social data collection and analysis.

But there is considerable question about how to select from among the hundreds of pieces of social information one could collect in any community without any guiding theory or set of principles. Sheldon and Freeman,[9] for example, have suggested that

> Evoking the economic analogy and proposing the develop-ment of social indicators that parallel economic indicators is confusing and in part fallacious. Despite its weaknesses and limited rigor, economic theory provides a definition and the specifications of an economic system, and the linkages are at least hypothesized, if not empirically demonstrated, between many variables in the system . . . Although some social scientists have proposed similar usefulness for social indica-tors . . . there is not even a reasonable anticipation. There is no social theory, even of a tentative nature, which defines the variables of social system and the relationships between them . . . Yet, without the guidance of theoretical formulations concerning significant variables and their linkages, one can hardly suggest that there exists, even potentially, a set of measures that parallel the economic variables.

Accordingly, most social indicators have been chosen inductively rather than deductively. By analyzing the full spectrum of information available about any community, it has been possible to identify specific variables over time and to eliminate highly redundant ones. As a consequence, social scientists have been able to select a small set of social indicators and apply them to any community at periodic intervals. For example, the Urban Institute[10] has proposed fourteen aspects of the quality of life and for each aspect has selected one best indicator. The fourteen aspects include poverty, indicated by the percent of low-income households; unemployment, indicated by the percent unemployed; racial equality, indicated by the ratio of non-white unemployment rate; mental health, indicated by suicide rate; health, indicated by infant mortality rate; traffic safety, indicated by traffic death rate; air pollution, indicated by the air pollution index; income level, indicated by per capita income; housing, indicated by the cost of housing; social disintegration, indicated by the narcotics addiction rate; community concern, as indicated by per capita United Fund contributions; public order, indicated by draft rejection rate; and citizen participation, indicated by the Presidential voting rate.

It is instructive to examine this list in some detail. First, the fourteen aspects of quality of life were not deductively identified from any theory. They are simply a thoughtfully selected list. Other groups could well have chosen a somewhat different list. Second, each indicator is quantitative and readily available in most communities. Indeed, it might appear that one selection criterion was an indicator's availability. Third, the indicators clearly bear different degrees of closeness to the variables they purport to index. Thus, while the indicators of health or income level seem straightforward enough, using draft rejection rate to index education or suicide rate to index mental health seems far more open to debate. Fourth, there is undoubtedly some redundancy among the indices, and the list can probably be shortened. For example, it is likely that poverty, income level, and housing are highly intercorrelated and that one indicator can serve for all three. But until such time as social indicators are derived from a theory of society or a theory of community, there is little alternative to being quite pragmatic about their selection. A variety of statistical procedures are available to locate independency and redundancy, and subsequent research can indicate utility.

Other lists of social indicators have been produced. A United Nations expert committee, concerned with measurement of "level of living"[11] proposed twelve categories: health, food and nutrition, education, conditions of work, aggregate consumption and savings, transportation, housing, clothing, recreation and entertainment, social security, and human freedoms. These twelve categories were subsequently collapsed into seven: nutrition, shelter, health, education, leisure, security, and environment.[12] In Denmark, the list includes such categories as children and family, social welfare, manpower and labor conditions, and leisure time activities. In France, the categories for which data are currently being collected include life expectancy, health protection, old people's place in society, employment trends, role of education, adaptation to change, social mobility, distribution of national wealth, utilization of income, urban development, and patterns of time-utilization.[13]

In a recent American publication,[14] the first to issue statistical time series data under the general heading of social indicators, information is organized around eight so-called social concerns: health, public safety, education, employment, income, housing, leisure and recreation, and population.[15]

The National Institute of Mental Health has developed a social area analysis program to identify areas with differing potentials for mental health and related problems.[16–18] As in the case of the Urban Institute, easy availability of data has played an important role in the selection of variables. The NIMH social area demographic profile variables are grouped into seven categories: (1) social rank, including measures of economic, social, and educational status; (2) life style, including such dimensions as family status, family life cycle, and residential life style; (3) ethnic status; (4) residential stability; (5) feminine careerism; (6) social area homogeneity; and (7) high risk populations, such as school dropouts, working mothers, and disabled populations. The demographic profile system is designed to make it possible for each community mental health center in the United States to understand a variety of demographic aspects of its community in order to facilitate need assessment and program planning.

These lists have much in common, yet each emphasizes certain aspects of the social condition and deemphasizes others. In reviewing these various sets of social indicators, Oborn[7] suggests that

> The various categorizations of social indicators according to subject area . . . are based on normatively selected areas of human needs, and while it is conceivable that one list of categories could be universally agreed upon, it is doubtful whether such agreement would ever take place or whether it is important that it should.

Three characteristics appear to be of nearly universal interest—(1) general health (sometimes including mental health and nutrition), (2) education, and (3) social welfare and public safety. It would be useful to give examples of specific measures suggested for each of these three. These examples are taken from the 1973 publication of the U.S. Office of Management and Budget. General health measures include specific measures of life expectancy, disability, and access to medical care. Examples of measures of life expectancy include life expectancy at birth, life remaining at ages 30 and 50, and infant mortality rate. Disability measures include days of disability per person per year, admission rates into mental hospitals and into nursing homes, and injury rates. Measures of access to medical care include extent of health insurance and personal confidence in ability to obtain good health care.

Measures of education include high school graduation rate, reading achievement, college entrance rates, and number of degrees awarded. Examples of measures of social welfare and public safety include persons below the poverty income level, substandard housing units, violent crimes, crimes against property, and persons afraid to walk alone at night.

Two points should be made about these examples. First, while these indicators are both objective (life expectancy at birth) and subjective (personal confidence in ability to obtain good health care), they are all presented in quantitative terms. The point is that there is no reason why subjective attitudes or opinions cannot be assessed in reliable and quantified form. The second point is that in most cases, but not all, it is clear how indicator changes are to be interpreted, that is, one would like to see an increase in life expectancy, a decrease in infant mortality rate, etc. But other indicators are more equivocal. Is a decrease in nursing home or mental hospital admission rate a good or bad sign? Is it a good sign if there is no difference in reading comprehension or mathematical skill between high school graduates and those who terminate their formal education prior to graduation?

## PROBLEMS WITH SOCIAL INDICATORS

One general area of difficulty in the social indicator approach to the analysis of community structure and community need has already been mentioned, namely the absence of a persuasive theory of community. Without such a theory it is impossible to know whether a complete or even an adequate set of indicators has been chosen.

A related concern is how changes in indicator magnitude over time should be interpreted. If unemployment rises from 8 percent to 9 percent, few would see this increase as anything other than an indication of a growing problem. If the body temperature goes up in a person already feverish, it is difficult to interpret that change as good news. But social indicator changes are not that easily interpreted. An increase in the number of days lost from work because of illness or injury could signal a decrease in the health status of the employed population. But it could also indicate a liberalization of sick leave policies.[9]

More fundamental is the issue of validity: the degree of correspondence between an abstract concept and the procedures employed for its measurement. There is considerable criticism about the validity of certain social indicators. For example, in discussing measurement in the field of education Cohen[19] has stated:

> When we survey the volumnious, yet unsuitable, data now available for assessing the products of education, we must conclude that practically none of it measures the output of our educational system in terms that really matter (that is, in terms of what students have learned).

As another example, while health-related expenditures are a frequently used index of health status, Bell[20] suggests that

> No one can say with any precision, what kind of correlation exists between various expenditures on health and actual state of the nation's health.

The authors of *Toward a Social Report*[6] suggest that

> Many of our statistics on social problems are merely a by-product of the informational requirements of routine management. This by-product process does not usually produce the information that we most need for policy or scholarly purposes, and it means that our supply of statistics has an accidental and unbalanced character . . . We have measures of death and illness, but no measures of physical vigor or mental health. We have measures of the level and distribution of income, but no measures of the satisfaction that income brings. We have measures of air and water pollution, but no way to tell whether our environment is, on balance, becoming uglier or more beautiful. We have some clues about the test performance of children, but no information about their creativity or attitude toward intellectual endeavor.

In a recent critical review of health status indicators, Goldsmith[21] asserts that definitions of health are ambiguous and imprecise, that the purposes of health status indicators need to be clarified, and that most currently used measures are inadequate. In developed countries, general measures of mortality are no longer useful because of the vastly decreased contribution of infectious disease to the overall mortality rate. Infant mortality rate, the most popular of all indices of mortality, is of limited reliability and not particularly useful as a health indicator in developed countries. Measures of morbidity (illness) are even more difficult to interpret because of problems of definition (How sick is sick?), problems of reliability, and extraordinary variation in different cultural and ethnic groups for the same apparent clinical condition.[22]

Access to medical care, as has already been mentioned, is indexed by such measures as extent of health insurance coverage, expenditures for health services, and degree of personal confidence in the ability to obtain good health care. Yet none of these gets at the fundamental question: do people in need of medical care get it? A new approach has been proposed by Taylor, Aday, and Anderson. These authors developed a measure based on the differences between the number of visits to a physician for a set of 20 symptoms that actually occurred to a sample population and the number of visits that a panel of physicians indicated is appropriate for these same symptoms. The authors found that

> Non-whites, rural farm people, the poor, and those who have no usual place to go for medical care . . . have less access to care than would be judged appropriate . . . (and that there is) possible "over-utilization" among certain groups such as children and people who see specialists as their regular source of care.[23]

Finally, the literature suggests that social indicators are used mainly to guide policy decisions and to aid in social program evaluation. Yet it is these two uses, according to Sheldon and Freeman, which are least easily defended. With regard to the use of social indicators in forming policy decisions, they state:[9]

> It would be foolish to argue against the use of indicators in program planning and development, or to expect their employment to disappear as a means of influencing politicians and their electorates. But it is naive to hold that social indicators in themselves permit decisions on which programs to implement, especially that they allow the setting of priorities. The use of data to make a case either already decided on other grounds or one that inevitably is going to be determined by political rather than "objective" considerations— whether or not it is in a good cause—is a weak basis for the indicator effort. Priorities do not depend on assembled data. Rather, they stem from national objectives and values and their hierarchical ordering.
> In short, when used for purposes of setting goals and

priorities, indicators must be regarded as inputs into a complex political mosaic. That they are potentially powerful tools in the development of social policy is not to be denied. But they do not make social policy development any more objective. Advocates of policy can strengthen their position by citing hard data and so can critics of those policies. In a situation where all sides have equity of resources to gather, interpret, and communicate indicator information, it could be argued that social indicators can serve to develop a more rational decisionmaking process in social policy development. But this is unlikely to be the case very often and in instances of unfair competition indicators are essentially a lobbying device.

The notion that data is selectively used to support a point of view and that competing factions should have equal access to data sources is important. It is reminiscent of the same concept in the legal profession, namely, that the adversary system works best when both sides have access to equally qualified legal staff. In both instances, when access is not equal, the process is corrupted. With regard to the use of social indicators for program evaluation, Sheldon and Freeman suggest that:[9]

> Concurrent with the movement to promote social indicators, there has developed a strenuous effort on the part of key individuals in and outside of government to estimate the gains that are derived from the initiation and expansion of different types of preventive and rehabilitative action programs. The terms "evaluation research" and "cost benefits analysis" now are common jargon among a vast number of such practitioners, planners, and politicians. The rationality of being able to estimate the benefits of expenditures of money, time, and manpower is virtually incontestable, and the utility of knowing whether existing and innovative programs work clearly is desirable.

> The empirical situation however is that there have been but a handful of respectable evaluation studies of social action programs: There simply are not very many crafts-

manlike evaluations of national programs, and there is increasing dissatisfaction with the failure to document by careful research the current massive programs now underway to improve the occupational, educational, mental and physical health status of community members. As a consequence, there is the temptation to argue for social indicators as a substitute for experimental evaluations. The fact of the matter is, however, that social indicator analyses cannot approximate the necessary requirements of sound design in order to provide for program evaluation.

Investigators who have thought about the problems of evaluation generally agree that there is no substitute for experimental research that differentiates between the effects of treatments and programs on the one hand and of extraneous contaminating factors on the other. Experimentally designed evaluations often are not possible because of resistance to the requisite random assignment of persons to different treatment groups. Thus, there is a turning to efforts of evaluation through statistical controls or "systems analyses."

The use of indicators to evaluate programs would require one to be able to demonstrate, via statistical manipulations, that programs determine the outcome measured by the indicators rather than other factors "causing" the results. There is no possibility at the present time of meeting the requirements of controlling for contaminating variables with available statistics that may be regarded as indicators, at least ones that cover large groups of individuals. In order to locate and identify factors that may be contaminating, knowledge of the determinants and interrelationships between determinants is required. Information is not available in many fields of social concern to do such analyses well, either on an empirical basis or a theoretical one.

But social indicators can be used for (1) improved descriptive reporting, (2) analytical studies of social change, and (3) actuarial prediction of the future. Even these objectives for the analysis of community characteristics and their changes, however, can only be met if measures are carefully chosen, reliably gathered, and more skillfully analyzed.

## Conclusions

The social indicators movement provides a strategy for identifying health needs that can potentially be of very high significance. Its usefulness is presently limited by the inadequacies of a theory of community and how its attributes impinge upon individual and group functioning; and by a seemingly irresistible tendency to use data collected for other purposes in the development of specific indicators. Yet currently collected information is underutilized, and before new measures requiring further increases in cost are designed, we should insist upon better use of available information. But, as this chapter has suggested, if social indicators are to achieve their optimal usefulness in need assessment and health services delivery system planning, there will probably need to be greater consideration of what problems we are trying to solve and what exactly we need to find out to approach their solution.

## Notes

1.  Maguire, C. Some principles in the evaluation of educational programs. *Mental Health Continuing Education in the West*, 1974, *1*, 21–28.

2.  Spencer, H. *The study of sociology*. New York: D. Appleton, 1882.

3.  Bauer, R. (Ed.) *Social indicators*. Cambridge, Mass.: M.I.T. Press, 1966.

4.  Wilcox, L.D., Brooks, R.M., Beal, G.M., & Klouglan, G.E. *Social indicators and societal monitoring: An annotated bibliography*. San Francisco: Jossey-Bass, 1972.

5.  Sheldon, E.B., & Parke, R. Social indicators. *Science*, 1975, *188*, 693–699.

6.  U.S. Department of Health, Education and Welfare. *Toward a social report*. Washington, D.C.: U.S. Gov't Ptg. Office, 1969.

7.  Oborn, P. T. *Review of the literature on social indicators.* Denver: Social Welfare Research Institute, University of Denver, 1972.

8.  Kahn, A. J. *Theory and practice of social planning.* New York: Russell Sage Foundation, 1969.

9.  Sheldon, E. B., & Freeman, H. E. Notes on social indicators: Promises and potential. *Policy Sciences,* 1970, *1,* 97–111.

10. Editors. Measuring the quality of life. *New Human Services Newsletter,* 1971, *1,* No. 4.

11. United Nations. *International definition and measurement of standards and levels of living.* New York: United Nations, 1954.

12. Drewnowski, J., & Wolfe, S. *The level of living index.* Report No. 4. Geneva: United Nations Research Institute for Social Development, 1966.

13. U.S. Senate Committee on Labor and Public Welfare. *Toward a social report.* Washington, D.C.: U.S. Gov't Ptg. Office, 1969.

14. U.S. Office of Management and Budget. *Social indicators.* Washington, D.C.: U.S. Gov't Ptg. Office, 1973.

15. Rossi, P. M. Community social indicators. In A. Campbell & P. E. Converse (Eds.) *The human meaning of social change.* New York: Russell Sage Foundation, 1972.

16. Redick, R. W., Goldsmith, H. F., & Unger, E. L. *1970 census data used to indicate areas with different potentials for mental health and related problems* (NIMH Mental Health Statistics Series C, No. 3 USPHS Publication, No. 2171) Washington, D.C.: U.S. Government Printing Office, 1971.

17. Goldsmith, H. F., Unger, E. L., Rosen, B. M., Shambaugh, J. P., & Windle, C. D. *A typological approach to doing social area analysis* (NIMH Mental Health Statistics Series C, No. 10) USPHS Publication Office, 1975.

18. Rosen, B. M., Lawrence, L., Goldsmith, H. F., Windle, C. D., & Shambaugh, J. P. *Mental health demographic profile system description: Purpose, contents and sample of uses* (NIMH Mental Health Statistics Series C, No. 11) USPHS Publication No. (ADM) 76–263. Washington, D.C.: U.S. Government Printing Office, 1975.

19. Cohen, W. J. Education and learning. *Annals of the American Academy of Political and Social Science,* 1967, *373,* 79–101.

20.   Bell, D., (Ed.) *Toward the year 2000: Work in progress*. Boston: Beacon Press, 1967.

21.   Goldsmith, S. B. The status of health status indicators. *Health Services Reports*, 1972, *87*, 212–220.

22.   Zola, I. Culture and symptoms: An analysis of patients' presenting complaints. *American Sociological Review*, 1966, *31*, 615–630.

23.   Taylor, D. G., Aday, L. A., & Andersen, R. A social indicator of access to medical care. *Journal of Health and Social Behavior*, 1975, *16*, 39–49.

# Chapter 9

# CLIENT ANALYSIS*

## Who are Your Potential Clients and What Do They Need

*Janet Scheff*

Human services include health, education, and welfare at the least. A broader definition might also consider employment, public order, private and public insurance, housing, and/or recreation. Obviously this chapter cannot analyze or even describe all or even most of these sectors. Instead I will emphasize health care as an example that is relevant to other sectors in terms of the major question: who are your potential clients and what do they need?

A historical perspective of health care is given in the first part of this chapter. The second and third parts, describing the client analysis† method and relating both it and need assessment to social planning, take a more general approach to human services.

*The original title of this presentation was "The Use of Client Utilization Data to Determine Social Planning Needs." This new title is based on the author's chapter in Proceedings of 25th Anniversary Conference, Department of City and Regional Planning, University of Pennsylvania, 1978.

†The term *Client Analysis* does not imply a focus on clients alone. Rather, it refers to a context in which clients are affected. In NIMH-supported research for 1979–81, the author labels this method *access analysis*.

## HISTORICAL PERSPECTIVE (THE HEALTH CASE)

Two concepts have dominated health planning in the past: adequacy and coordination. Between 1880 and 1920, hospitals in the United States grew thirty-fold, and total population only doubled. Estimates of bed requirements were based upon crude expectations of morbidity.[1] Now, over 50 years later, bed requirements are calculated in much the same manner.[2] During the 1930s the concept of functional coordination of hospitals and physicians within a region was introduced. The U.S. Hospital Survey and Construction Act of 1946, commonly known as the Hill-Burton Act, wed these two concepts by requiring as a prerequisite for federal aid for facility construction a state plan based on a survey of extant facilities and on a regional hierarchy of base and intermediate hospitals and health centers.

In the past decade, facilities planning has developed sophisticated methods for dealing with adequacy and coordination. The methodologies used parallel industrial location theory, making estimates of number, types, and locations of facilities based on access and cost. The Hill-Burton program, however, has not accomplished a close-knit health system, largely because it relies on informal relations and voluntary cooperation between the various providers of health care.

In the 1950s and 1960s, the problem of coordination was again raised by various voluntary, hospital, and governmental groups, resulting in the formation of some hospital councils. A few regional agencies called "318 agencies" because of their relation to that law, were formed by hospitals in response to the Hill-Burton program. Fearing direct federal intervention, some providers tried to organize local voluntary agencies. These councils have had three purposes: to encourage cooperation in direct patient care, to engage in cooperative action in solving community problems, and to coordinate capital planning and fund raising.[3]

A large number of these councils were formed in response to the scrutiny and criticism by community leaders and donors to hospital fund drives of conflicting capital programs. Composed of the brokers who provided and raised capital and the service suppliers (i.e., hospital administrators), they attempted to rationalize the demands upon the donors and to assure that each hospital got a piece of the pie. In general, they have had little success, for they "are in most cases loose federations, with prime decision-making power remaining in local units."[4]

The Community Health Service Act of 1961 provided operating funds for area-wide agencies, and the Hill-Harris amendments to the Hill-Burton Act in 1964 provided more money for planning. In 1963, the Public Health Service issued Procedures for Areawide Health Facility Planning, which included such agency purposes as determining and projecting needs for services, facilities, and personnel; providing information and guidance for decision-makers; and developing systematic procedures for project evaluation.

In 1965, the Regional Medical Program, or RMP, was established to attack certain specific health problems. It departed somewhat from traditional planning in that area plans, not institutional plans, were based on local needs and were directed by advisory councils composed of representatives of voluntary groups, planning agencies, public agencies, universities, and the public in addition to providers. Thus the control base extended beyond just the providers. However, the law made it clear that the programs were to be run through existing health services and were not to interfere with the "existing patterns of professional practice of medicine."[4]

The federal laws passed during 1965 and 1966, that is, the Regional Medical Program and the Comprehensive Health Planning Program, were explicitly tied to planning for improving the delivery of personal health services. During that same period, the law known as "Medicare for the Aged and Medicaid for the Indigent" was passed. Its impact was primarily upon reimbursement methods for hospitals, nursing homes, and physicians' fees. To this date it only affects planning indirectly. Nevertheless, by vastly expanding the number of potential and actual clients, it has heightened utilization and interest in both planning and evaluation.

It did become obvious that coordination and planning must incorporate all participants: non-Department of Health agencies and even representatives of the citizenry as potential services users. This broader approach was embodied in the Comprehensive Health Planning Program, also known as the Partnership for Health Act. The planning envisioned by this law included all sectors of government and all providers and consumers interested in general health, mental health, and environmental health planning. This context appeared better able to create a rational, user-oriented health system. Obviously, the methods chosen for planning within this political context were potentially a major determinant of the probability of achieving this new health care system.

Also, in 1965 in New York State and in the nation, reports were coming in on ways to control hospital costs. In the late 1960s, Article 28 (passed in 1965) was amended, and by June 1970 responsibility had shifted to the Public Health Council. Thus, the New York State Department of Health was given comprehensive responsibility for developing and administering the state's health and hospital planning functions for hospitals and related facilities and for services provided therein. Specifically: (1) the applicant had to obtain all approvals and consents and (2) the Commissioner had to be satisfied as to the public need for the construction at the time and place and under the circumstances proposed. This was planning with clout. This, then, was the certification of need.

Unfortunately, neither this article, and its amendments, nor subsequent legislation has truly changed the direction of health planning toward a rational, user-oriented health system. Even the community-based decentralization of both health and mental health centers has not increased community participation in assessing and providing for health needs.

But, during the past decade, public officials, administrators, and social scientists in a variety of disciplines increasingly have focused on the emerging social demands that public programs be linked directly to identified and assessed human need. It is in this context that the client analysis method is described since it can identify and assess utilization and rejection of offered services by a target population and, on the basis of these findings, establish or alter programs designed to reduce community need.

## CLIENT ANALYSIS

During the past few years, there are indications in the health field that client analysis can both fill an information gap and pay more than lip service to consumer representation via the first steps of comprehension and relevance. As a writer in the *American Journal of Public Health* stated:[5]

> The theme of the demands for popular control that is most favorable to the planners is that 'the appropriate decision makers are the members of society, acting directly and through their representatives . . . Planners, as such, have no special competence for the making or guidance of social policy, but only for the enlightenment of the process by which it is made. Enlightenment may, of course, be achieved in many ways: by intuitive insight, by scientific discovery, by systematic and orderly arrangement of data, by quantification, by criticism, and so forth. What all these ways have in common is that none endows the planner with any special responsibility for determining social policy or with any special wisdom for guiding it.'
> This doctrine is a difficult one for health planners to accept; yet, if they do not, they may be lucky to encounter this doctrine rather than be faced with a popular demand that denies them any role at all. The problem is the development of institutions that will make professional planners responsive to popular control, while still enabling them to enlighten the process of public decisions.

Thus, the recognition of the problem calls for development of new ways to relate the delivery of health services to community needs. We will now examine how client analysis can be used to bridge this gap between community input and professional reception of that input. The method constructs a set of parameters in which need assessment of health delivery systems can be evaluated and thus improved.

The general context of the client analysis method is emphasis on people as the hallmark for planning and democratic decision making. This emphasis on the individual as the unit of analysis can take several forms. First, the impact of activity must be measured in terms of specific individuals; second, the suppliers and the client populations (i.e., target populations) cannot be seen as faceless institutions; and third, the affected individual's preferences and choices are central to the planning effort.

Most obviously, the incorporation of client analysis forces planners to look beyond the physical, the economic, and the rational in terms of both objectives and constraints. Bolan and Nuttall[6] suggested during this past decade, as did Davidoff and Reiner[7] and Faludi[8] over 20 years ago, that the nature of the public agenda, the character of the decision system, and the components of the system are dependent on the interactions of each of these elements and their subunits. The tensions in the decision-making process (as well as their normative nature) are central to planning. They are more precisely accounted for through instruments such as client analysis.

We refer to the sum of these individuals within a specific territory as the target population. The target population can be broken down systematically into many components (Figure 9–1). Subdivisions may occur along several dimensions. Demo-

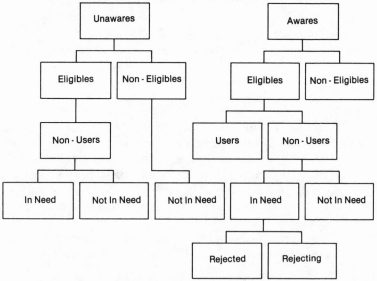

**Figure 9–1 Types of target area populations**

graphic age cohort estimates and measures of population-at-risk have been incorporated in human services planning for decades. But more analytic or critical parameters are also required to understand the communication distortions and gaps that result in program biases.

These gaps are seen most clearly when we survey a target area and discover that only some subpopulations are aware of the existing program. How does this occur? For example, everyone does not read the newspapers where a program announcement may have been placed. If we first divide the population into those who are aware and those who are not aware, determine whether each sample is eligible or not and which of the eligibles are users, and then proceed to describe who is and is not in need within existing program limits, we have a new approach to operationalizing self-selection and rejection within the limits of program regulations and program actions.

This concern with communication can be shown in the following step-by-step description of the client analysis method:

1.  A statement of what the law establishing each program commits the government to do; that is, a statement of what benefits or services are to be provided for what part of the population.
2.  An estimate of the past and present size of the population for which the services of the program (or programs) are by law intended. For convenience this population is called the client population (which is parallel to "target population").
3.  An estimate of the past and present number of those actually receiving the services provided, labeled the program's clients.
4.  A comparison, to the extent possible with existing data, of the characteristics of clients with the characteristics of the total client population. While secondary sources are the most economical, it may be necessary even at this early stage to engage in field work. The client population, for example, may not be identified by the census or other data sources nor by estimates based on relevant investigations elsewhere.
5.  A statement of the conditions under which each pro-

gram's services are offered, including policies and practices of the administering agency, which restrict the number of clients to some fraction of the client population. In general, the number of clients of a program will be limited by: (a) *selection standards*, limits on who can participate based on explicit requirements and procedures of the agency administering the program; (b) *standards of service*, including location and other convenience factors of the program; and (c) *preferences*, the knowledge and inclinations of members of the client population. Further investigation related to the last step is necessary where the findings of earlier studies indicate that the characteristics of the clients differ substantially from those of the client population. This investigation is a study of the conditions under which services and benefits of each program are offered and received. The easiest aspect is content analysis of written documents, such as manuals of procedure and administrative regulations. Less simple would be application of the activity analysis (developed and applied in a need assessment context to hospital use and rejection by Stuart Chapin[9]) or, though it is less operational, the goal-oriented approach to planning developed by sociologist-planner Herbert Gans,[10] which involves observation, analysis, and generation of empirical indicators.

6.  Projections utilizing the basic demographic and economic projections, on which much of the planning of the government is based, of the future size of the client population of the program.

7.  Projections of the probable future number of actual clients of the program, based on past trends in selection standards and standards of service and upon the past responses of the members of the population to these trends.

These projections provide a frame of reference that may be thought of as the basic data for long-range planning. They are based primarily on projections of national income, population, and labor force.

As can be seen, this frame of reference represents an analysis of ongoing developments. It provides the most suitable starting point since it rests on forces and potentialities already under way. In this sense, the projections do not represent facts or goals; they are taken as today's best estimates of tomorrow.

## SOCIAL PLANNING

Client analysis involves a conceptual base and method for determining human service planning needs and the evaluation of the actual service delivery mechanisms. The main purpose thus far has been to identify the necessary steps in client analysis as well as to demonstrate its utility for need assessment. A brief history has been provided as background on the lack of real or at least people-oriented planning in the health sector. In the final section, the concept of social planning will be introduced to demonstrate that people-oriented or social planning can be effective planning. Social planning, which falls between and therefore connects social policy and social programming, is happening via such need assessment approaches as client analysis.

A central role of client analysis and need assessment in social planning is in analyses of the impacts of particular government programs on particular populations. Planners can approach this question from two directions: that of abstraction or that of empirical studies of particular kinds of public policies to determine their distributive effects.

The client analysis approach to social planning makes two assumptions that should be explicated. One is that the services and resources provided are worth getting. The usefulness of the services is not fundamentally questioned. Client analysis centers on the distributive question of who receives the program offering. If the question of usefulness or relevance is introduced, new questions emerge. The second assumption is that it is desirable to concentrate more resources and activities on those subpopulations hardest to affect.

Discussion of client analysis can all be encompassed within the conceptual framework of need assessment. Need assessment itself is now recognized generally as a planning function. It is asserted here, however, that if client analysis and associated approaches to need assessment are considered the major social planning function, then the significant contribution of social planning is providing feedback. Thus, we also have at the policy level instruments that can directly effect distribution of public resources and thus societally effect redistribution.

On the other hand, social planning may be dichotomized into social programming and societal planning. Here the connection is lost between the information provided by methods such as client analysis or need assessment and the development and use of strategies, models, theories, or plans for social change. Obviously social indicators and other information provided by need assessment or client analysis are not sufficient for societal planning (or social policy) or even for social programming, but they (need assessment and client analysis) are necessary for more rational policy and programs.

The position taken here is that: (1) *post hoc* assessment of program performance and client analysis of program reception allows determination of goal-seeking behavior and (2) goal changes can be induced from observation of changes in behavior when the process of client analysis is repeated over time. This induced value assessment can be relevant to achievement of goal-directed behavior as well as to the study of need. The planner can therefore more precisely gauge and influence the community members' capacity for making social choices.

Social planning is an effort to focus on the human element of action. The social planner constructs a model of society and plans for development. Meanings of the two terms, society and development, vary among and within planning specialities, but some elements recur. Society is the universe or map on which the planner works. Development is both the goal and the means toward achieving change to which the planner contributes. Neither society nor development is a static concept, and neither is necessarily dependent on planning. Both require macrocosmic as well as microcosmic analysis for planning or even for understanding. Neither is simply social or simply economic or simply physical. While planning practice and its scientific rationale (social and physical sciences) are so divided today, it must be recognized that this division is an analytic device and not a representation of reality.

The content and principles of social planning involve units of analysis that vary by the scale of interaction—individual, family, community, region, nation, world; by the effects of the interaction (i.e., the type of change or nonchange that results); and by the source and degree of intervention. The social planning activity reflects both the changing tasks and skills of planners over the past decades and the societal changes. Six basic concepts of social planning are identifiable:

1. *Sectoral planning or welfare planning.* Planning for a particular sector of society where traditional criteria of efficiency provide no guide constitutes the first class of social planning. Planning for health and welfare programs and facilities are good examples. In addition to the absence of clear-cut measures of merit, or objectives, there are distinct and serious measurement problems in this field. For example, is the unit of analysis simply the number of clients served or can one enter with qualitative considerations? Also, externalities and third party benefits (as well as costs) abound. A second characteristic of these sectors (particularly health and welfare) is that their planning must perforce be conducted with a view to a mix of operating as well as capital expenditures, with the former often significantly greater than the latter. A given level of performance can usually be attained by several alternative mixes, some more and some less labor or service intensive. It is essential that the social planner learn the substances of these sectors with great emphasis on their development over time.

2. *Human resources planning.* Partly as an outgrowth of this type of planning, we note increasing efforts and respectability given to the planning of education systems, labor training and retraining, leisure time activity, etc.—in short, human resource planning. The unit of analysis is people: hence the occasional designation of these efforts as social planning. There appears to be a close linkage to planning for depressed areas, either training for migration or changing the locational advantage of the area. Since education is but one facet

of the human resource plan, this type of social planning (as is true for the first category) involves study of health, welfare, recreation, and other services and facilities that directly bring people into contact with publicly and privately supplied services. Obviously the welfare and human resource approaches are connected. Obviously also, all members of society require one emphasis or the other, but the total society requires them both.

3. *Planning as a residual from physical and economic planning.* Given a fairly well-defined scope for physical planning (equivalent largely to the tasks assigned to urban planners) and for economic planning (corresponding on the whole to the work of national planners), there still remains scope for planning activity. The residual function has, on occasion, been labeled as social planning. Again, there is considerable overlap with the work of the social planner under definitions 1 and 2 above. However, this residual notion embraces other tasks; for example, the determination of appropriate growth rates for subsystems of the nation. Thus such regional criteria as equalization of welfare, and their implementation, come to be incorporated in this category. Inasmuch as, traditionally, economic planning is keyed to system criteria of performance (such as maximizing gross national product), physical planning lacks the metric to be sensitive to alternative planning projects of the type which affect per capita income differentials over time between regions. Increasingly, the label *social planning* is attached to the steps by which physical or economic goals are achieved. This may well involve manipulation of the population through education, persuasion, and provision of incentives or sanctions. Social planning is the sum of these. The study of the reaction to the implementation of physical and economic goals likewise can fall under this rubric.

4. *Social planning as the techniques by which societal objectives are identified.* The most recent label for this type is social policy planning. The social planner is, then, the value technician. His or her task is to pinpoint possible objec-

tives for the system with which he or she is associated and assess their relationships and their relative costs and benefits (the pricing structure itself might be proper scope for this activity).

The impact of the alternate objectives on various institutions, classes, and subsystems might appropriately be studied in terms of feasibility, compatibility, etc. This last type has been termed societal planning by some. We might also include advocate planning which assumes distinct interests for subgroups of society) and which requires preparation and promotion of different plans. Advocate planning is occasionally supported through public funds. But it is normally in conflict with public planning agencies which assume that there is a single public interest which the planning agency by definition expresses.

5. *Social planning as providing the theoretical base that planning requires.* It should be noted, in caveat, that a majority of planners insist that planning is practical and therefore practice, not theory, is necessary. For this theoretical approach, however, the terms "societal planning," "transactive planning," and "socially oriented development planning" as well as simply "planning" have been employed. I do not mean to imply that these terms describe identical concepts. I will, however, try to distinguish their basic theoretical differences: (a) a few consider it possible to develop a theoretical base for planning that is independent of the social sciences; (b) some see planning as theoretically synthetic, that is, synthesizing in a unique way theories from one or more of the social sciences; and (c) some apply a theory or theories of one or more social sciences without adaptive efforts since, in sociologic terms, planning is an institution that is not unique. A prime example of the first type can be seen in the behavioristic choice theory concept of planning developed during the 1950s by Davidoff and Reiner,[7] Faludi,[8] and earlier in Paul and Percival Goodman's *Communitas*.[11] Work by John Friedman in *Retracking America*[12] provides an example of the second synthesizing approach as does

Herbert Gans' work, but Gans in most of his efforts is closer to the third approach.[13,14] Another approach, conceptually distinct but resembling Gans in its reliance on social science theory, is that of a few economists who enlarge and often basically alter the process and the substance in dealing with the larger picture but who base their work totally on economic theory. This last type is most explicitly seen in socially oriented development planning as shown in applications of welfare economics.

6. *The interactionist approach to planning.* This approach, if admitted to the planning profession at all, is considered a type of social planning. It assumes that persons affected by a plan or program must be primary participants in the planning process. Indirectly, this is achieved by client analysis and similar approaches. Directly, it is achieved most satisfactorily through community study and in those cases where the entire community is organized through advocacy planning. We will say more on these approaches later on.

These six categories of social planning obviously include overlapping sets, and the definitions indicate the complexity and enormity of the subject. These types of social planning serve well to identify differing emphases in social planning endeavors. But identification of the type of emphasis is not enough to comprehend the total job of the social planner. In other words, the social planner's job is a complex one, and to understand it we must be able to distinguish varying concepts of social planning.

Regardless of the type, overall social planning has two aspects: the societal aspect encompasses the goals and aims of the society while the sectoral aspect deals with subsidiary goals as instruments in achieving societal goals and aims. In the societal sense, social planning means planning for the development of the society, for the improvement and equalization of the welfare of its members. Social planning requires:

1. The analysis of the society into its component social groups and into the detailed social framework within which these groups interrelate.

2.  The articulation of goals and aims of each of these groups, their priorities, and potential conflicts, both internally and externally.
3.  The operationalizing of the goals into specific sectors and geographic areas.
4.  The programming for sectoral activities to reach towards those goals.

Two of the most important social planning methods that deal with all four of these requirements are community study and client analysis.

In summary, this chapter proposes a method that is useful for need assessment and for social planning, and that can be specifically applied for relating recognized public preferences to actual government performance in the human services. This method, client analysis, supplemented by the community study approach, can have two major consequences. The first is increased knowledge (e.g., about the clients). The second may be change in the law aspects of program management. The client analysis method increases the capacity of the public to evaluate the action of its government and, via a feedback mechanism, the government's capacity to plan. These results are achieved through formal organization of program information and socioeconomic data in a manner that relates program mission to accomplishment. But in conclusion we should remember that just as the six categories of social planning, and the two levels (the societal and sectoral) are not discrete, so too any method for improving the planning process is not sufficient to the entire task. The potential importance of need assessment in linking service providers to communities should not be understated. The next task, however, is to link need assessment to a possible future which not only considers new alternative governmental policies but also stresses the support of existing, vital, informal processes in the community.

## NOTES

1.  Anderson, O. W. *The uneasy equilibrium.* New Haven, Conn.: College and University Press, 1968.

2. Public Law 89–749, P.L. 89–239, P.O. 75 (1046 and subsequent amendments).

3. May, J. J. Health planning: Its past and potential. *Health Administration Perspectives,* No. 5, Chicago: University of Chicago, Center for Health Administration Studies, 1967.

4. Blum, H. L. *Notes on comprehensive planning for health.* Berkeley, Ca.: Western Regional Office, American Public Health Association, 1967.

5. Feingold, E. The changing political character of health planning. *American Journal of Public Health,* 1969, *89*(5), 806.

6. Bolan, R. S., & Nuttall, R. L. *Urban planning and politics.* Lexington, Mass.: Lexington Books, 1974.

7. Davidoff, P., & Reiner, T. A. A choice theory of planning. In A. Faludi (Ed.), *A reader in planning theory.* New York: Pergamon Press, 1973, pp. 11–39.

8. Faludi, A. (Ed.) *A reader in planning theory.* New York: Pergamon Press, 1973.

9. Chapin, F. S., Jr. *Human activity patterns in the city.* New York: John Wiley, 1974.

10. Gans, H. J. *Recreation planning for leisure behavior: A goal-oriented approach.* Unpublished Ph.D. dissertation. University of Pennsylvania, 1957.

11. Goodman, P., & Goodman, P. *Communitas* (2nd ed., rev.). New York: Vintage Books, 1960.

12. Friedman, J. *Retracking America.* New York: Doubleday, 1973.

13. Gans, H. J. *The urban villagers.* New York: The Free Press of Glencoe, 1962.

14. Gans, H. J. *More equality.* New York: Random House, 1974.

*Chapter 10*

# THE USE OF THE FIELD SURVEY TO ESTIMATE MENTAL HEALTH NEEDS

*George J. Warheit*
*Roger A. Bell*

## INTRODUCTION

Need assessment methods based on field surveys rely on the collection of data from a sample or entire population of persons living in a community. Most commonly, schedules or questionnaires designed to elicit information regarding health, social well-being, and patterns of care are administered to respondents by phone or personal interview.

The gathering of information by means of surveys has had a long history. In ancient times, surveys designed for the enumeration of populations were often used for purposes of taxation, the procurement of laborers for work projects, or military duty. By contemporary standards, the design and methodologies employed by Caesar's census takers may suffer from comparison with those employed by the Bureau of the Census. Early Roman censuses were, nonetheless, effective sources of valuable information, and to this day surveys represent one of the most useful tools for collecting information about individuals. Obviously, the survey approach is not the only useful method for obtaining need assessment data. However, when done correctly, it is an excellent one for assessing needs and care patterns and for evaluating and restructuring service programs. This chapter outlines the rationale and processes related to survey development, conduct, and utilization. The focus is on field surveys designed to measure mental health needs and services although many of the issues involved in doing surveys are generic. The design and method issues discussed reflect our own field experiences. Over the past decade and a half we have completed a number of field surveys designed to assess the mental health needs and utilization patterns of persons in the general population. To date we have interviewed over 6,000 randomly selected adults (18–65 years of age) in a number of different counties in the Southeastern United States. Many of the findings have been reported in the literature.[1–6]

A review of the methods and findings from these and other field surveys of an epidemiologic nature is beyond the purpose of this chapter and will not be presented. Dohrenwend and Dohrenwend, however, have systematically summarized 88 studies of psychological disorder conducted throughout the world, and a careful reading of their work is recommended for those interested in the substantive findings of these studies and in the theoretical and methodologic issues associated with them.[7]

We are cognizant of the theoretical and methodologic problems encountered in conducting field surveys designed to assess mental health needs and urge those conducting such surveys to familiarize themselves with the theoretical obstacles likely to be encountered.[8–14]

It has been suggested by Lapouse and others that until the basic problems related to the definition and diagnosis of mental illness are solved, field studies will have little value as guides for planning services.[13] We do not believe this is necessarily so. Our experience has shown it is possible to assess the need for mental health services without becoming entangled in the morass of problems associated with field survey case identification procedures. We have not resolved this issue but rather have avoided it by using a statistical-normative approach to the distribution of symptoms and functioning levels among various social and demographic groups. We constructed items, scales, and indices that are amenable to scoring, summarization, and analysis in keeping with statistical models of central tendency. We assume psychiatric symptoms are randomly distributed and identify as needers those whose symptom and/or dysfunction levels are one or more standard deviations above the mean for the population from which the sample was drawn. As a check for the utility of this method, we have interviewed approximately 500 psychiatric patients and compared their scores with those of nonpatient community samples. Patient scores are statistically different from those scoring at or below the mean among community samples; conversely, patient scores are generally similar on these measures to those in the high scale score ranges.[15]

From a methodologic perspective, it has been argued that field surveys are of limited value as a need assessment method because of the problems of validity and reliability. This criticism is very important and cannot be ignored. However, the problem of response reliability is not unique to field surveys. The individual's answers must be considered with caution any time information is reported about themselves or others. The problems of memory span, accurate recall, verbal skills, response set, and social desirability are always present and need to be considered by those who are going to make judgments on the basis of the information received.

At another level, field surveys are characterized as being too complex to conceive, too costly to conduct, and beyond the technical competence of most agencies. And, as such, it is argued, they should not be considered viable options when an agency is contemplating the initiation of a need assessment program. It is true that surveys, particularly very large ones, designed to measure prevalence or incidence are more difficult to define, conceptualize, and operationalize than any of the other assessment approaches. However, not all surveys need to be large and complex; neither do they need to be prohibitively expensive, even for agencies with limited staff and financial resources. This is especially true when previously developed and tested methods and materials are used as a basis for the survey. And because we believe field surveys are the most scientific and, hence, the most accurate of all assessment approaches, we urge they be considered seriously by those contemplating a need assessment program. The utility of surveys is particularly enhanced when they are used with target populations previously identified by agency records, key informant judgments, and/or social indicator analyses.

## DESIGN

### Introduction

Need assessment based on field surveys is initiated, as all good research is, by defining the objectives and operationalizing the concepts by which valid information can be most practically and economically obtained. It is important to emphasize that the cooperation of other organizations and agencies in the community should be enlisted before the survey is begun. Their involvement during the early development stages encourages a more comprehensive approach to the questions being asked, and although there are size limitations to a survey instrument, often questions can be included that are meaningful to a wide variety of agencies in the community. Questions that might be included are those dealing with the utilization of services, consumer satisfaction, and perceived impediments to care. The inclusion of other community organizations and agencies can also assist in gaining legitimation and cooperation. Local medical societies, Chambers of Commerce, consumer protection groups, and law enforcement agencies often facilitate entry into respondent's homes and/or encourage their participation. This is an important consideration.

Another reason for including other organizations in the planning process is that many of the needs revealed by the survey will be beyond the response capabilities of any one agency. Referrals, consultations, and the development of cooperative service programs designed to meet these needs will be facilitated by enlisting the guidance and support of the community's human service agencies at the beginning of the planning process.

### Data Gathering Techniques

The three most common techniques used in surveys to gather information are (1) the telephone interview; (2) the mailed questionnaire; (3) the personal interview. Although methodology of each is somewhat different, their basic format is the same. Each employs a series of questions asked of respondents. The questions are designed to elicit information about an individual's mental and physical health, medical history, use of human service agencies, self perceptions of health and social needs, family problems, and other related topics.

Each method has individual characteristics that strongly influence the following:

1.  Sampling procedures.
2.  Length of the questionnaire or interview schedule.
3.  Format in which the questions can be asked, recorded, and coded.
4.  Amount of time required to complete it.
5.  Nonreturn or refusal rates.
6.  Costs in time and dollars.
7.  Validity of the findings.

The steering committee will need to weigh each technique carefully and select the one most compatible with their interests, capabilities, and resources.

## Preparing the Items

The items selected for inclusion in the instrument ought to have a direct relationship to the specific goals of the program. The tendency is to include a great many items because they are interesting; this should be avoided for a number of reasons. A large number of items that have no immediate relationship to the project's goals tend to fragment the questionnaire-schedule so that it loses its structural integrity; the cost of gathering and analyzing the data is increased; and, by overburdening the respondent, the response rate may be reduced, a condition that tends to limit the validity of the findings.

After the items have been selected, decisions regarding their format must be made. The format influences response rate, the cost of gathering, coding, and processing the data, and, importantly, the types of statistical methods one can use in analyzing the results. For example, *open-ended questions,* when asked in a mailed questionnaire, take more time to answer than *fixed alternative types,* a fact which tends to increase the nonresponse rate. These types of questions also complicate coding procedures and limit modes of analysis. A limited number of open-ended questions may be asked but these ought to be clearly stated, easily answered, and near the end of the questionnaire.

The issue of which type of question to ask is related to the debate over *structured* versus *unstructured* questionnaires-schedules. This controversy has gone on for a long time and remains largely unresolved. Our own preferences are strongly in favor of the structured format for several reasons. First, it reduces interviewer contamination, produces a greater homogeneity of responses, and provides data that are more efficiently coded and analyzed. In addition, structured items take less time to answer; this permits the asking of more questions in a given time period. And, importantly, the structured formating with fixed alternative items greatly expands the types of statistical tests that can be used for analysis. Data gathered by unstructured schedules or questionnaires with a great many open-ended items rarely meets the assumptions required for statistical tests based on ordinal or interval scaling characteristics.

## Selecting the Sample

Once the type of survey has been selected and the items prepared and put in a questionnaire or interview schedule, a sample must be drawn. Some of the issues related to sampling methods are:

1.  How large should the sample be?
2.  Which sampling technique should be used?
3.  How can a sampling frame be prepared?
4.  How will the data be analyzed?
5.  What are the relative costs associated with each of the sampling procedures?

The answers to these questions will be determined largely by the type of survey. Ultimately, sample selection depends on the information needed: the unit for analysis, that is, individuals, households, etc.; the type of data gathering technique used; and the size it must be to adequately represent the population from which it is drawn. Standard statistics books provide detailed procedures for sample selection. In addition our manual, *Needs Assessment Approaches: Concepts and Methods* offers many helpful suggestions.[16]

## Obtaining the Data

The next step is to obtain the data. Procedures for doing this will be determined largely by the type of survey selected. Telephone and mail surveys are less complex than personal interviews. In all three, however, there are a number of ways to permit successful data collection. For example, advance publicity much like that associated with preparations for the community forum will facilitate the process.

Once this important groundwork is completed, the committee can begin the data gathering process. This includes recruiting and training interviewers and, in the case of mail surveys, assigning persons to tasks related to sending questionnaires.

## Coding the Data

After the data have been collected, they must be coded before they can be tabulated. The type of coding procedures used will depend on the format of the questions, that is, whether they are fixed alternative or open-ended, the structure of the instrument, the amount of information obtained, and the mode of analysis planned. When the instrument is structured, contains few open-ended questions, and has been designed for direct coding, the task of transferring the answers is relatively simple although it must be done with caution. Unstructured instruments with large numbers of open-ended questions are difficult to code because the responses have to be listed and placed in categories before they can be coded or tallied. This difference highlights one of the basic advantages to structured instruments and forced option responses.

## Preparing the Data for Analysis

The least technical way to prepare most data for analysis is tally sheets that can be set up so the questions are listed along with their response alternatives. Each answer is then manually tallied and the totals summed. Such an approach permits some elementary statistical analysis; for example, averages and standard deviations can be computed for the total sample and for its various subgroups such as age, race, sex, and income. Although it would be possible to do a number of more advanced statistical tests with the aid of a calculator, the process is so cumbersome and time consuming it is usually not advisable, particularly when there is a big sample or a large number of items in the instrument. In the overwhelming majority of cases, it is more advisable to transfer the data to cards or magnetic tape for computer analysis. With the aid of a computer, tremendous areas of analysis are opened which, perhaps many will find surprising, are often less expensive than manual tabulations. The availability of computer services is so commonplace almost all agencies can utilize this method of analyzing research data.

## PRESENTING THE FINDINGS AND RECOMMENDATIONS

The final stages of a survey consist of presenting the findings and making recommendations.

The findings can be presented in a variety of ways, such as summary tables, charts, diagrams, and statistical tests. Once again, the exact mode of presentation depends on the objectives of the study, the design of the survey, and the structure of the questions. Complex statistical analyses have their place, but they should be presented to audiences that understand the assumptions and implications of such techniques. For most groups, descriptive summaries, charts, diagrams, and other visual aids will probably be far more effective. The selection of which method to use is best determined by the purposes of the study, the nature of the data, and the character of the audience.

It is important to include as part of the final report a list of priorities and recommendations for action; and, as noted earlier, such lists ought to include time-cost estimates. A check list that summarizes activities for those using field surveys as a needs assessment method is found in Appendix A.

## Conclusions

This chapter has discussed the use of field surveys as a method for assessing needs and services utilization patterns. A brief discussion outlined the basic steps involved in conducting an assessment survey. It is worth noting again in closing a point made earlier in the discussion on surveys, their relative complexity, costs, and effectiveness. Our experience suggests surveys are practical and economically feasible when used in conjunction with other assessment approaches. The reasoning behind this judgment is that rates-under-treatment, community forums, key informants, and social indicator data can be obtained at modest cost. These methods, however, tend to lack the scientific precision possible with field surveys. Therefore, we recommend surveys be used with social, demographic, and/or geographic groups identified as being at greater than average risk by other more manageable and economic methods. This process reduces the sample size because it focuses on a target group already distinguished on the basis of need, and, in addition, it permits researchers to cross validate the findings from two or more different approaches.

## Appendix A

*Activities Check List*

1.   The committee will need to begin by describing carefully the overall objectives of the study. On the basis of these objectives, it will develop the concepts appropriate to the inquiry and operationalize these goals and concepts by preparing a design-methods outline to guide them throughout each stage of the process.

2.  The population to be studied needs to be "identified" and an appropriate sample prepared.

3.  The items for the questionnaire/schedule will need to be decided upon; their format and design will also need to be determined in the light of the objectives of the study, the unit for analysis, and anticipated methods of analysis and presentation.

4.  Interviewers will need to be recruited and trained, or, in the case of a mailed questionnaire, letters will need to be prepared for mailing.

5.  An extensive program of publicity should be commenced just prior to the initiation of the survey.

6.  Appropriate agencies in the community that can "legitimate" the study should be contacted and apprised of the program. It is often important to inform law enforcement agencies, Chambers of Commerce, medical societies, and other community groups that a survey is being conducted since they are sometimes called by citizens who have been selected as respondents/informants in the survey.

7.  A system for coding, punching, and analyzing the data will need to be decided upon and put into effect during the survey.

8.  Once the data is gathered, it must be analyzed for presentation.

9.  The findings need to be presented along with a list of recommendations for action. These recommendations are more effective when they are listed in a rank order based on their priority. A time-cost estimate should accompany the list of recommendations.

## Notes

1.  Schwab, J. J., McGinnis, N., & Warheit, G. J. Social change, culture change and mental health. *Excerpta Medica,* 1971, Series 274, Symposium 12, 703–709.

2.  Schwab, J. J., Warheit, G. J., & Holzer, C. E. Suicidal ideation and behavior in a general population. *Diseases of the Nervous System,* 1972, *33*(11), 745–748.

3. Warheit, G. J., Holzer, C. E., & Schwab, J. J. An analysis of social class and racial differences in depressive symptomatology: A community study. *Journal of Health and Social Behavior*, 1973, *14*(4), 291–299.

4. Warheit, G. J., Holzer, C. E., & Arey, S. A. Race and mental illness: An epidemiologic update. *Journal of Health and Social Behavior*, 1975, *16*(4), 243–256.

5. Warheit, G. J., Arey, S. A., & Swanson, E. Patterns of drug use: An epidemiologic overview. *Journal of Drug Issues*, 1976, *6*(3), 223–237.

6. Warheit, G. J., Holzer, C. E., Bell, R. A., & Arey, S. A. Sex, marital status and mental health: A reappraisal. *Social Forces*, 1976, *55*(2), 459–470.

7. Dohrenwend, B. P., & Dohrenwend, B. S. Social and cultural influences on psychopathology. *Annual Review of Psychology*, 1974, *25*, 417–452.

8. Blum, H. L. *Planning for health*. New York: Behavioral Publications, 1975.

9. Siegel, L. M., Attkisson, C. C., & Cohn, A. H. *Mental assessment: Strategies and techniques*. National Institute of Mental Health Report. Washington, D.C.: U.S. Government Printing Office, 1974.

10. Mechanic, D. Problems and prospects in psychiatric epidemiology. In E. Hare & J. K. Wing (Eds.), *An international symposium on psychiatric epidemiology*. London: Oxford University Press, 1970.

11. Kosa, J., Albert, J., & Haggerty, E. On the reliability of family health information. *Social Science and Medicine*, 1967, *1*, 165–181.

12. Crandell, D. L., & Dohrenwend, B. P. Some relations among psychiatric symptoms, organic illness, and social class. *American Journal of Psychiatry*, 1967, *123*(12), 1527–1537.

13. Lapouse, R. Problems in studying the prevalence of psychiatric disorder. *American Journal of Public Health*, 1967, *57*, 947–954.

14. Dohrenwend, B. P., & Dohrenwend, B. S. The problem of validity in field studies of psychological disorder. *Journal of Abnormal Psychology*, 1965, *70*(1), 52–68.

15. Kuldau, J. M., Warheit, G. J., & Holzer, C. E. *Health opinion survey valid for needs assessment*. Paper presented at the annual meeting of

the National Council for Community Mental Health Centers, Atlanta, Georgia, 1977.

16.    Warheit, G. J., Bell, R. A., & Schwab, J. J. *Needs assessment approaches: Concepts and methods* (DHEW Publication No.(ADM) 77–472). Washington, D.C.: U.S. Government Printing Office, 1977.

*Chapter 11*

# SURVEYING THE QUALITY OF LIFE IN THE COMMUNITY*

*Alex Zautra*
*Nancy Kochenowicz,*
*Darlene Goodhart*

Many approaches may be used to assess the quality of life (QOL) in communities. For instance, social indicators can monitor changes in the objective conditions of community life, such as unemployment and poverty,[1] and describe environmental features, such as housing density and spatial organization, thought to influence QOL.[2] Behavior settings can map the staffing patterns of economic, health, recreational, and even aesthetic settings in the community.[3] A different type of assessment procedure is the focus of the present study: the use of subjective information from community members as the primary measure of QOL.

One of the most important standards for judging QOL in the community resides in the subjective evaluations of the "goodness" of life as reported by community members themselves.[4] In-depth survey interviews can ask residents about their activities and values, their satisfactions, and their crises to assess individual

*The authors wish to express appreciation to the Research, Evaluation and Planning Bureau of Behavioral Health Services of Arizona for their assistance.

needs and to study well-being in the community as a whole. By providing direct information about the life experiences of persons living under different social conditions, subjective data also put "flesh" onto objective indicators of well-being. This chapter reviews some of the major research on these subjective indicators of QOL and gives an example of a community survey of life quality conducted in the Tri-City (Tempe, Mesa, Chandler) region of Arizona.

## RESEARCH ON LIFE QUALITY

### A Positive Mental Health Perspective

A positive mental health perspective provided a framework for investigating QOL.[5] From this perspective, QOL has two separate components: adjustment and life satisfaction. Adjustment relates to the person's effectiveness in diminishing, avoiding, or adjusting to painful life experiences. Satisfaction, on the other hand, refers to the individual's ability to find positive and growth-producing experiences. Research further suggests that, except under extreme circumstances, adjustment may be unrelated to life satisfaction, meaning the ability to cope with adverse situations may not be associated with one's ability to derive satisfaction from life experiences.[6,7] Two major influences on satisfaction and adjustment are (1) the actual events the person experiences and (2) her or his social and personal resources that may influence the impact of life events on evaluations of QOL. Thus, a framework for judging QOL should include assessments of both adjustment and life satisfaction, as well as the events and resources that affect these two QOL components.

### Components of Adjustment

*Stressful Life Events.*    Initial research into measuring the effects of life events was guided by Selye's[8] notion of adaptation that views all life events, both positive and negative, as stressful and therefore as threats to the person's psychological well-being. Both the number and magnitude of stressful events that occur may predict the degree of stress experienced by the organism. Psychological adjustment depends on the degree to which major changes in one's life do not occur, since change taxes the individual's adjustive capacity and requires the expenditure of energy to rebalance upset psychological forces. Many investigations have suggested that stressful life events may lead to adjustment difficulties.[9,10] Research in community settings has also found the occurrence of stressful life events to be associated with decrements in psychological well-being.[11]

The occurrence of stressful life events, however, does not always lead to adjustment difficulties.[11] The perspective of crisis theory[12] views both developmental and environmental changes as life crises that can either promote or hamper adjustment. An unsuccessfully resolved crisis brings psychological deterioration and impairs ability for future crisis management. A successfully resolved crisis, on the other hand, promotes adjustment and improves skills for coping with future crises. Effective crisis resolution is thought to depend on the adequacy of personal and social resources available to the person under stress.[13]

*Personal and Social Resources.*   Of the many personal and social resources that can promote adjustment, social support from family, friends, and other relationships has received considerable empirical attention. Social support may supply information and trusted feedback needed to act in a stressful environment, and provide a refuge from overwhelming stressful situations.[14] Several studies have found that differences in adjustment depend on available social support. Nuckolls, Cassel, and Kaplan[15] found that women with many stressful life events who reported few social resources had significantly more medical complications with their pregnancies. Other researchers have attempted to identify more specific functions of socially supportive relationships thought to facilitate adjustment such as intimacy[16] and "social integration," defined as shared values, goals, and activities.[17]

Other resources that may influence adjustment include previous successes in coping with life stress[12] and social and marital status.[18] Alternatively, personal characteristics like a propensity to blame others for one's misfortunes may constitute a "negative resource."[19,20]

*Adjustment Criteria.*    Adjustment has typically been assessed using measures of psychiatric symptoms that mental health professionals have rated to be indicative of psychopathology.[21] Assessing rates of psychopathology in the community with these methods has been a major focus of epidemiologic studies of mental disorder.

Epidemiologic studies attempting to estimate "true prevalence" of mental disorder have been beset by a host of difficulties, however. First, sizable variations in rates of disorder (from less than 1 percent to greater than 65 percent) have been reported, suggesting there are many unresolved questions regarding what constitutes a "case" of mental disorder.[13] A second difficulty is the presence of systematic biases in reports of symptoms due to cultural norms governing self-disclosure and tendencies to give socially desirable responses.[22]

Despite these difficulties, epidemiologic studies have led to many advances in the measurement of adjustment, particularly with those aspects of adjustment that are sensitive to social conditions,[23] as well as stressful life events such as marital discord, job loss, and other social disruptions.[14,24]

## Components of Life Satisfaction

*Positive Life Experiences.*    In addition to adjusting to painful life experiences, people seek to enhance their life satisfaction, to develop competence, and to perceive themselves as active agents controlling their own lives.[25] Events that lead to satisfaction and competence are thought to involve some intrinsically satisfying task or activity.[7] For instance, Herzberg summarizes numerous studies that show that when employees report exceptionally good work experiences they talk about times in which they were actively involved in a satisfying task and/or in receiving positive feedback about their accomplishments. The correlates of subjectively rated positive (and negative) events from the Holmes and Rahe *Social Readjustment Rating Scale*[26] have also been studied by Zautra and Simons.[27] In that study, positive events were associated with higher ratings of QOL and more frequent reports of positive feelings.

*Personal and Social Resources.* Personal and social resources may mediate the effects of positive life experience on satisfaction and happiness. Social resources, in particular, have been studied as correlates of perceived QOL, and efforts have been made to identify specific characteristics of social relationships possibly responsible for higher QOL. Brim[28] found that high degrees of assistance, value similarity, and concern in one's social relationships were significantly associated with avowed happiness. Participation in social activities is also considered an important social asset that contributes to happiness, [6,29] even for psychiatrically disturbed individuals.[29]

Personal characteristics such as interests, values, and skills may be highly instrumental in determining what is regarded as satisfying. For example, individuals with different interests and values would probably seek different kinds of life experiences to promote their own satisfaction and QOL.[30] Personal values, in addition, seem to help mold the meaning of life events and determine their impact on the individual's QOL.[31]

*Criteria for Satisfaction and Happiness.* A number of researchers have investigated the structure of people's perceptions of their life satisfaction and happiness and have developed methods to measure these components of QOL. In nationwide surveys, Andrews and Withey[32] and Campbell, Converse, and Rodgers[33] have developed comprehensive QOL inventories measuring level of satisfaction and dissatisfaction in various life domains such as family, work, leisure, and health. Overall QOL is thought to depend on the degree of satisfaction in these specific life concerns.

Avowed happiness has also been investigated and measured as a component of QOL.[6] Bradburn,[6] who developed the *Affect*

*Balance Scale (ABS)* to measure avowed happiness, suggests that happiness is composed of two feeling states, positive and negative affect, and that the measured discrepancy between these two states is the best predictor of overall happiness. Research on the *ABS* has repeatedly shown the two affects to be statistically independent from one another[32] and related to different aspects of well-being. Adjustment appears to be at least partly measured by Bradburn's[6] *Negative Affect Scale,* and satisfactions assessed to some degree with the *Positive Affect Scale* of the *ABS.*

## THE TRI-CITY STUDY

The previous research suggests that aspects of QOL can be assessed to aid in our understanding of psychological well-being in the community. A survey was designed to study QOL by selecting (and at times developing) measures that might tap major components of satisfaction and adjustment including positive as well as stressful life events, social support resources, and subjective ratings of psychological well-being. The Tri-City area of Arizona was selected as the site for this investigation.

### The Tri-City Sample

This survey was conducted with 537 residents of Tempe, Mesa, and Chandler, Arizona, who were selected using probability sampling techniques[34] to represent the approximately 250,000 residents in the area. (The completion rate was 85 percent of the originally selected sample.) The area's population is highly diverse. The surveyed group paralleled this population and contained college-aged students at Arizona State University in Tempe, suburban residents of both Tempe and Mesa, a Mexican-American subcommunity, and a large retirement population. The survey respondents were preselected by address, contacted by letter, then visited in their homes where the interviews took place. Twenty-five graduate and undergraduate students of Arizona State University conducted these interviews, which averaged approximately an hour and fifteen minutes in length.

*Survey Measures†*

*Life Event Measures.*    The occurrence of major events in the person's life was expected to be an important influence on ratings of QOL. One of the most popular inventories of life events is the *Social Readjustment Rating Scale* (SRRS).[26] The *SRRS*, however, has been criticized for failing to differentiate between the outcomes of positive and negative events.[35] For the Tri-City survey, major revisions of the *SRRS* were made to (1) clarify ambiguous items, (2) add more positive events to tap satisfactions, and (3) allow respondents to subjectively rate the outcome of the event. For example, items such as "changes in number of family arguments" were clarified to ascertain whether the frequency of family disputes had increased, decreased, or both. Also, 21 new positive events were selected from a sample of "exceptionally good" life experiences reported by community residents in a previous survey,[36,37] lengthening the life events inventory to 65 items. For each item, residents were asked to indicate first, if the event had occurred during the previous year, and, second, whether the *outcome* was positive or negative. Although this inventory could be scored in a variety of ways, two measures appeared to be particularly valuable as QOL indicators. These were the number of events rated as having negative outcomes, which might be indicative of potential adjustment problems, and the number of events with positive outcomes, which might signify occasions contributing to life satisfaction.

*Social Support Resources.*    In addition to major events, QOL may also depend on the nature of a person's social support network. Several measures were selected for the survey. The *Social Participation Scale*[29] was used to assess the extent of residents' formal and informal social contacts. Also, an inventory

---

†The entire survey schedule is not presented here. Only measures that summarized important indicators of life events, social resources and subjective ratings of psychological well-being are described. Copies of the entire inventory may be obtained from Alex Zautra, Department of Psychology, Arizona State University, Tempe, Arizona 85281.

to measure *Resources* asked respondents to indicate the degree to which each of a variety of potential resources helped them in times of trouble. These resources included religious beliefs, family, friends, and professional advice. Another measure, *Responsibilities,* was designed to assess the person's level of social integration. Residents were asked to identify their responsibilities to themselves, their families, their work setting, and five other areas of concern.[36] Scores consisted of the number of responsibilities mentioned in different life domains.

*Negative Resources.*   Some types of concerns pertaining to one's relations with others were thought to have an adverse impact on QOL. This was assessed with a measure of *Family Problem History,* asking if an immediate family member had experienced personal problems that required professional mental health care, led to legal difficulties, and/or led to difficulties in school during the last five years. The total number of problems mentioned constituted the score on this measure. Also, a measure of *Blame* assessed the degree to which the person tended to blame him- or herself and others for misfortunes. Blaming has been suggested to be a mechanism for maintaining maladjusted behavior.[19] Characteristics of the person as well as poor fit between the person and his or her social environment may contribute to "blaming" behavior. Residents were asked, "In your experience, which of the following are often (sometimes or never) the *cause* of you being less than completely happy with your life?" These potential "causes" included financial troubles, the government, one's self, one's family, lack of opportunity, one's employer, one's social life, and "other." The score on this *Blame* measure was the mean of ratings for the eight causes.

*Psychological Well-being.*   Measures of life events and social support are valuable QOL indicators in their own right. However, QOL can also be assessed more directly by obtaining subjective ratings of the respondent's level of psychological adjustment and life satisfaction. The satisfaction and adjustment indices were selected to provide comprehensive measures of community residents' evaluations of their QOL. Adjustment was assessed with the 22-item *Psychiatric Screening Inventory,*[21] that measures psychiatric symptoms such as loss of appetite, listlessness, worry, and sleeplessness. The Bradburn[6] *Negative Affect Scale,* that consists of five items asking whether the respondent recently felt restless, lonely, bored, depressed, and/or upset by criticism, also measured adjustment. The two measures of satisfaction included the Bradburn *Positive Affect Scale,*[6] consisting of five items to assess recently experienced pleasant feeling states (e.g., interest, excitement, and pride), and 16 items from the Andrews and Withey *Perceived Quality of Life Scale*[32] to appraise level of satisfaction with important life concerns such as family, work, leisure, income, community life, and one's personal life. In addition, a measure of overall QOL was obtained by asking residents, "How do you feel about your life as a whole?" twice during the interview. The mean score of the two responses to this question served as an indicator of overall QOL.

The *Positive Affect Scale* has the advantage of being independent of measures of adjustment and may therefore be helpful in identifying the particular life events and social resources that add to satisfaction as well as maladjustment. Although the perceived QOL items do not measure satisfactions separately from dissatisfactions (each of the items asks for evaluations along a single dimension of "delighted" to "terrible"), the scale does provide ratings of well-being in important areas of life, which may assist in defining the QOL problems of community members with greater specificity.

### Selected Findings

The first question we asked about the data was how measures of adjustment were related to indices of satisfaction. We began by examining positive affect. Based on previous research, we anticipated that positive affect would not be associated with adjustment measures but would contribute to ratings of satisfaction.[32] The findings supported these expectations. *Positive affect* appeared to be uncorrelated with adjustment as measured by *negative affect* ($r = .04$, $df = 525$, $p > .20$) and psychiatric symptoms ($r = -.03$, $df = 525$, $p > .20$). *Positive affect,* however, did seem to contribute to ratings of important satisfactions regarding self, family, job, health, and leisure (i.e., amount of fun) and was moderately correlated with overall QOL, as shown in Table 11–1. *Negative affect,* as expected, was correlated with psychiatric symptoms ($r = .38$) and was negatively associated with ratings of satisfaction with self, leisure, family life, and overall QOL. Thus, *negative affect* appeared to signify poorer adjustment and, concomitantly, a less favorable QOL.

A second major question asked of the data was how the measures of life events and social resources were related to ratings of satisfaction and adjustment. We anticipated that life

**Table 11–1    Correlations Among Ratings of Life Quality**

|  | Positive[+] Affect | Negative[+] Affect |
|---|---|---|
| **Perceived Life Quality Measures*** |  |  |
| Overall life quality | .41 | -.23 |
| Yourself | .29 | -.29 |
| Family Life | .20 | -.21 |
| Income | .16 | -.17 |
| Amount of fun | .29 | -.32 |
| Health | .22 | -.12 |
| Job | .21 | -.13 |
| Things done with family | .18 | -.17 |
| Spare time use | .16 | -.23 |
| House or apartment | .15 | -.16 |
| Community | - | -.11 |

*Only ten of the most representative perceived life quality items are listed here.

[+]$\underline{p}<.005$ for all correlations listed. Only statistically significant correlations are given ($\underline{p}<.05$).

events in general would prompt reports of more negative affect and psychiatric symptoms. In line with a positive mental health perspective, however, we expected positive events to have the added effect of enhancing the positive components of QOL. The results showed that events subjectively rated as having negative outcomes were associated with more *negative affect* ($r = .33$, $df = 525$, $p < .001$) and slightly less *positive affect* ($r = .11$, $df = 525$, $p < .005$). Negative events were also related to reports of more psychiatric symptoms ($r = .35$). Positive events, on the other hand, were associated most strongly with *positive affect* ($r = .33$). However, positive events also appeared to be related to reports of *negative affect* ($r = .20$) and to psychiatric symptoms ($r = .14$). It appears that all life events may be disruptive and contribute to adjustment problems for some people. Positive events, however, seem to have the added effect of augmenting some of the positive aspects of well-being.

Relationships between social resources and most QOL measures emerged as anticipated. The number of responsibilities reported was associated with greater *positive affect* ($r = .26$), as were more *resources* ($r = .28$) and *social participation* ($r = .18$). However, contrary to our expectations, the respondent's *resources* did not reduce her or his reports of *negative affect* or psychiatric symptoms. Apparently, one's adjustment needs are not affected by the extensiveness of one's social assets. One negative resource we studied was blaming. Residents who tended to blame a great deal also reported more *negative affect* ($r = .38$) and psychiatric symptoms ($r = .32$). Scores on the *Blame* scale were further related to negative events ($r = .31$), suggesting that some of their attributions may have been justified. Even when controlling for the effects of these life events, however, blaming contributed significantly to the prediction of maladjustment. Interestingly, this measure was also related to positive events ($r = .24$) but did not affect positive ratings of well-being. This suggests that a blaming style may be independent of the satisfactions one receives from life. A history of family problems ($r = .22$) and low *social participation* ($r = -.14$) also increased *negative affect* somewhat.

Figure 11–1 presents the proportion of variance accounted for in *positive affect* and *negative affect* by measures of life events

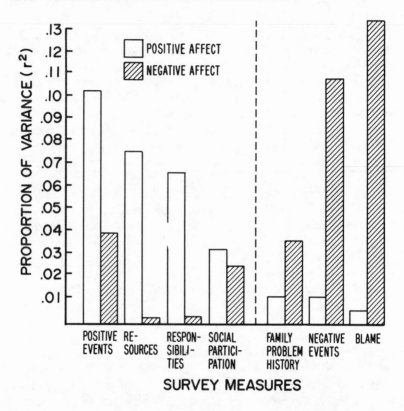

**Figure 11–1   Proportion of variance accounted for in positive and negative affect by survey measures. (Dotted line separates those measures correlated with positive affect from those correlated with negative affect.)**

and social resources. Clearly, the correlations are relatively modest, ranging from less than 1 percent to slightly over 13 percent of the variance accounted for. Figure 11–1 also shows that measures that influenced *negative affect* tended to be unrelated to *positive affect* and vice versa, signifying that the two affects may be associated with different kinds of life experiences and social resources. This pattern of findings lends further credence to the notion of studying the positive and negative components of QOL separately. Aspects of the life experience that lead to satisfaction may be qualitatively different from those leading to good adjustment.

These findings provide some preliminary support for the validity of residents' reports of their own QOL. The measures used in the survey have demonstrated consistent intercorrelations and appear to be sensitive both to major events in the person's life and to the quality of her or his social relationships. Two findings seem to be particularly striking. First, positively rated life events may have consequences that are both stressful and satisfying—a finding often obscured in studies assessing only adjustment outcomes.[38] Second, negative resources, especially blaming, may actually be detrimental. The harm in blaming may result from the fact that it more easily enables the individual to maintain poor adjustment rather than actively seek effective solutions to difficulties.[19] Just as society may play a major role in maintaining social inequities by "blaming the victim,"[39] so too many individuals contribute to their own problems by intensely blaming themselves and others for their misfortunes.

*Applications*

Data from studies like the present one may be applied in many ways. For example, this data may highlight the specific needs of persons within a given demographic group. One demographic group we are studying closely is the aged. From state service utilization records, we determined that these older residents (65+ years of age) were underutilizers of the mental health, alcohol, and drug abuse services offered by public agencies. Consistent with these low utilization rates, the older respondents in the Tri-City survey reported fewer problems of psychological adjustment. Their psychiatric symptoms, negative affect scores, and frequencies of stressful life events were significantly lower than those of younger residents. However, this group also reported significantly fewer positive life events and lower levels of positive affect. Thus, while older persons did not seem to be as troubled by adjustment problems, their QOL, as reflected in the frequency of their pleasurable feeling states and satisfying life experiences was considerably less favorable than that of younger respondents.

To examine these relationships further, we focused our attention on the responses of these senior residents to our life events measure. Of the items on this measure, those related to death seemed to be the only experiences occurring *more* frequently in the lives of older persons during the last 12 months. Death of a spouse and death of a close friend were reported, respectively, by 12 percent and 35 percent of those 65 years or older. These same events were reported by only 2 percent and 15 percent, respectively, of the total sample. Most other types of events, both positive and negative, occurred *less* frequently in the lives of senior members of the Tri-City community. While older residents had experienced fewer major frustrations (13 percent compared to 24 percent for the total sample), they also reported considerably fewer events that might mark instances of personal accomplishment and signify continuation of activities related to self-expression and personal growth. For example, 47 percent of the general sample stated they had learned a new hobby in the last year, but only 20 percent of persons over 65 claimed to have done so. There was also a sharp drop in the number of new friendships reported by older persons. About half of the total sample reported an increase in their number of friendships during the last year, but only about one third of the senior respondents claimed similar increases.

Findings such as these are suggestive of the type of services that could be provided to enhance the QOL of the senior residents of the Tri-City community. It is obvious from their scores on adjustment measures that this group would have little use for traditional mental health services. However, their responses to psychological indices of satisfaction strongly suggest that they could indeed benefit from services that provided them with greater opportunities to engage in pleasurable social and personal activities.

In addition to pointing out factors affecting the QOL of particular demographic groups, data from studies like the current one may also be helpful in highlighting the special needs of a given neighborhood or census tract. For example, we are taking a close look at certain census neighborhoods in the Tri-City area. One area that stands out is a small Southwestern-style ghetto contained within the boundaries of a single census tract. This area has a population slightly over 4,000, 87 percent of whom are Spanish speaking. About one-third of the residents are American- or Mexican-(Yaqui) Indian, and, at last count, around 50 percent of the families residing there are below the poverty level. In this census area, we expected our survey to find higher rates of psychiatric symptoms and stressful life events. Our results did not disappoint us. Of the 46 census tracts investigated, this area experienced the highest frequency of adverse life events (based on the stressful life events measure) and the highest symptom counts (a mean of 5.29 symptoms on the 22-item scale).

The rates of service utilization for this census tract (obtained from state records), however, matched neither the social indicator data nor our psychological indicators of distress. When we discovered these rates to be among the lowest of all census tracts studied, we suspected that the region was not only underserved, possibly due to language barriers, but that families were stubbornly refusing needed help because of self-imposed cultural barriers to service use. Nonetheless, when we looked further into our data, we found that, on the whole, residents of this region reported moderate to high levels of positive life events. As we discovered upon further analysis, these residents had managed to preserve a "sense of community" in which they felt they belonged and in which they shared common values (and hardships) with their neighbors.

This area is undoubtedly underserved according to all of our criteria of adjustment. However, an evaluation of the community's QOL from a perspective different from that typically offered by epidemiologic models reveals that this area has special positive features that cannot be ignored in understanding its mental health needs. Interventions intended to reduce residents' distress should be carefully designed so as not to unintentionally diminish the seemingly ample opportunities for positive experiences provided by this community.

These two examples illustrate the importance of obtaining subjective data from community members to identify both the special needs of certain groups as well as existing community resources that could be used to advantage by thoughtful planners. The present study further illustrates the importance of assessing the positive dimensions of community life. Had our primary focus been the traditional examination of forces hindering adjustment, we would have missed a great deal of valuable information about the life experiences of different community groups. We could have been (mis)led into believing, for example, that we could do little to enhance QOL for our elderly populations and that QOL in our Southwestern ghetto was so impoverished as to demand drastic measures. This rather limited understanding could induce us to allocate service resources in ways that would either fail to provide for the needs of certain groups and/or possibly interfere with the functioning of special preventive forces already operating. However, by identifying the degree to which both positive and negative aspects of QOL are present in the lives of community members, services could be distributed more effectively and equitably. In this manner, planners might be helped to avoid "brush fire" styles of service delivery that allocate resources hit-or-miss as needs happen to "flare up" among various constituencies in the community.

## SUMMARY

In this chapter, research is reviewed and a survey described for studying quality of life in the community. The survey adopts a positive mental health perspective that views both adjustment and satisfaction as contributors to life quality. Resident reports of adjustment and satisfaction were expected to be influenced to some degree by major life experiences and personal/social resources. A survey to measure these components of life quality was administered to 537 residents of a Tri-City region in Arizona. Based on correlational analysis, survey findings indicate that aspects of quality of life can be assessed, although incompletely, and that studying satisfactions separately from adjustment seems informative and valuable. Applications of this data for understanding the real-life problems of aged residents and members of a Mexican-American community suggest that a quality of life survey may have considerable utility as an aid to mental health planning.

## NOTES

1.    Liu, B. C. *Quality of life indicators in U.S. metropolitan areas: A statistical analysis.* New York: Praeger, 1976.

2.  Proshansky, H. M., Ittelson, W. H., & Rivlin, L. G. *Environmental psychology*. New York: Holt, Rinehart & Winston, Inc. 1970.

3.  Barker, R. G., & Schoggen, P. *Qualities of community life*. San Francisco: Jossey-Bass, 1973.

4.  Campbell, A., & Converse, P. Social change and human change. In A. Campbell & P. Converse (Eds.), *The human meaning of social change*. New York: Russell Sage Foundation, 1972.

5.  Jahoda, M. *Current concepts of positive mental health*. New York: Basic Books, 1958.

6.  Bradburn, H. M. *The structure of psychological well-being*. Chicago: Aldine, 1969.

7.  Herzberg, F. *The managerial choice*. Homewood, Ill. Dow Jones-Irwin, 1976.

8.  Selye, H. *The stress of life*. New York: McGraw-Hill, 1956.

9.  Holmes, T. H., & Masuda, M. Life change and illness susceptibility. In B. S. Dohrenwend & B. P. Dohrenwend (Eds.), *Stressful life events: Their nature and effects*. New York: Wiley, 1974.

10. Spilken, A. Z., & Jacobs, M. A. Prediction of illness behavior from measures of life crisis, manifest distress and maladaptive coping. *Psychosomatic Medicine*, 1971, *33*, 251–264.

11. Myers, J. K., Lindenthal, J. J., & Pepper, M. P. Life events and psychiatric symptoms. In B. S. Dohrenwend, & B. P. Dohrenwend (Eds.), *Stressful life events*. New York: Wiley, 1974.

12. Caplan, G. *Principles of preventive psychiatry*. New York: Basic Books, 1964.

13. Dohrenwend, B. P., & Dohrenwend, B. S. *Social status and psychological disorder: A causal inquiry*. New York: Wiley-Interscience, 1969.

14. Cassel, J. Social science in epidemiology: Psycho-social processes and "stress." Theoretical formulation. In E. G. Struening & M. Guttentag (Eds.), *Handbook of evaluation research*, (Vol. I). Beverly Hills: Sage Publications, 1975.

15. Nuckolls, K. B., Cassel, J., & Kaplan, B. H. Psycho-social assets, life crisis and the prognosis of pregnancy. *American Journal of Epidemiology*, 1972, *95*, 431–441.

16. Brown, G. W., Bhrolchain, M., & Harris, T. Social class and psychiatric disturbance among women in an urban population. *Sociology*, 1975, *9*, 225–254.

17.  Kochanowicz, N. *Social supports of crime and crisis victims.* (approximate title). Unpublished Masters Thesis, Arizona State University, Tempe, Arizona, 1978.

18.  Zautra, A., & Beier, E. Life crisis and psychological adjustment. *American Journal of Community Psychology,* 1978, *6,* 125–135.

19.  Beier, E. G. *The silent language of psychotherapy.* Chicago: Aldine, 1966.

20.  Bulman, R. J., & Wortman, C. B. Attributions of blame and coping in the "real world": Severe accident victims relate to their lot. *Journal of Personality and Social Psychology,* 1977, *35,* 351–363.

21.  Langner, T. S. Twenty-two item screening scale of psychiatric symptoms indicating impairment. *Journal of Health and Human Behavior,* 1962, *3,* 269–276.

22.  Klassen, D., Hornstra, R. K., & Anderson, P. B. Influence of social desirability on symptom and mood reporting in a community survey. *Journal of Consulting and Clinical Psychology,* 1975, *45,* 448–452.

23.  Dohrenwend, B. P. Sociocultural and social-psychological factors in the genesis of mental disorders. *Journal of Health and Social Behavior,* 1975, *16,* 365–392.

24.  Dohrenwend, B. S. Life events as stressors: A methodological inquiry. *Journal of Health and Social Behavior,* 1973, *14,* 167–175.

25.  DeCharms, R. *Personal causation.* New York: Academic Press, 1968.

26.  Holmes, T. H., & Rahe, R. H. The Social Readjustment Rating Scale. *Journal of Psychosomatic Research,* 1967, *11,* 213–218.

27.  Zautra, A., & Simons, L. S. Some effects of positive life events on community mental health. *American Journal of Community Psychology,* 1979, *7,* 441–451.

28.  Brim, J. A. Social network correlates of avowed happiness. *Journal of Nervous and Mental Disease,* 1974, *58,* 432–439.

29.  Phillips, D. L. Mental health status, social participation and happiness. *Journal of Health and Social Behavior,* 1967, *8,* 285–296.

30.  Rokeach, M. *The nature of human values.* New York: The Free Press, 1973.

31.  Dohrenwend, B. S. Social stress and community psychology. *American Journal of Community Psychology,* 1978, *6,* 1–14.

32. Andrews, F. M., & Withey, S. B. *Social indicators of well-being: Americans' perceptions of life quality.* New York: Plenum Press, 1976.

33. Campbell, A., Converse, P. E., & Rodgers, W. L. *The quality of American life.* New York: Russell Sage Foundation, 1976.

34. Sudman, S. *Applied sampling.* New York: Academic Press, 1976.

35. Houghs, R., Fairbank, D., & Garcia, A. Problems in the ratio measurement of life stress. *Journal of Health and Social Behavior,* 1978, *17,* 70–82.

36. Zautra, A., Beier, E., & Cappel, L. The dimensions of life quality in a community. *American Journal of Community Psychology,* 1977, *5,* 85–98.

37. Flanagan, J. C. A research approach to improving our quality of life. *American Psychologist,* 1978, *33,* 138–147.

38. Vinokur, A., & Selzer, M. A. Desirable versus undesirable life events: Their relationship to stress and mental stress. *Journal of Personality and Social Psychology,* 1975, *32,* 329–337.

39. Ryan, W. *Blaming the victim.* New York: Random House, 1971.

*Chapter 12*

# THE NOMINAL GROUP AS A TECHNIQUE FOR UNDERSTANDING THE QUALITATIVE DIMENSIONS OF CLIENT NEEDS

*André L. Delbecq*

## QUALITATIVE VERSUS QUANTITATIVE NEED ASSESSMENT

A good deal of the focus in the need assessment literature is on allocative planning, that is, the generation of data to determine the size of the client population and the amount of resources that should be directed toward client services. However, need assessment often encompasses not simply the identification of a population group in need of services but also the investigation of the qualitative character of client needs in order to facilitate the design of services to meet client needs.

For example, if an agency is interested in providing services to single parents (where the providing agency has not had prior experience in the delivery of these services), need assessment does not end simply with the identification of the number of single parents in a community. The agency must also understand the qualitative character of the need. What problems do single parents have? What dysfunctional consequences emerge as the result of poor coping with these problems? Unless a rich clinical understanding of client problems is coupled with data describing numbers and characteristics of clients, need assessment provides only limited direction for program and policy decisions. This chapter describes a technique for adding qualitative richness to need assessment where the nature of the problem is only vaguely understood.

## CLIENT PARTICIPATION IN NEEDS IDENTIFICATION

A fundamental value espoused by most providers of services is that clients should have the opportunity to define problems and needs in their own frame of reference, rather than having service providers "lay on" a definition of problems and solutions. The difficulty, of course, is to facilitate provocative client dialogue. It was precisely to structure client participation in defining needs that the nominal group technique (NGT) was developed. It originated as a mechanism whereby providing agencies could meet with panels of clients to elicit responses that accurately portrayed the character of clients' problems as defined by clients.

In every instance where we have compared the attributes that clients use to describe a problem with the descriptions given by providers of services, there has been a statistically significant difference between client and provider perceptions. It is not that providers are uninformed. Rather, because they are not themselves in the problem context and possess different skills and attitudes than clients, their perspective is always incomplete and skewed differently from clients. The challenge was to discover a technique whereby clients themselves could accurately portray their perspective.

Understanding the qualitative dimensions of problems is not easily accomplished by either interview or written surveys. Unless the survey designer is already well informed about all dimensions of user needs, client responses to a survey provide distributive information only about those problem attributes that the provider has preconceived. This chapter presents a useful group technique for problem exploration that can be combined with observation and unstructured interviewing for purposes of understanding the qualitative aspects of client needs: NGT.

## THE NOMINAL GROUP PROCESS

Let us imagine a situation where planners are concerned with providing services to single parents. Quantitative indicators show a substantial number of single parent households among the target population. Further, the data indicates ethnic, racial, geographic, and economic differences within the client group. Consequently, planners are concerned with understanding the qualitative nature of the problems faced by clients, in general, and the differences between subgroups. Then action recommendations can anticipate the character of clinical services to be provided to the different subpopulations. The planners adopt NGT as a means to explore the problem. The process can be described as follows.

Twenty or thirty clients are brought together for a meeting to discuss their individual and common problems that are the focal issues around which the new service program will emerge. The representative of the planning group opens the meeting by indicating the sincere interest of his organization in understanding the character of the client's problems so that his organization might better plan its program of services. He indicates that the purpose of the meeting is to understand problems, not to explore solutions. The planner then divides clients into groups of six to nine according to distributive characteristics (such as age, race, income) and has these small groups sit around tables. Each client is asked to list on a work sheet the problems he or she faces as a single parent. Each client spends the next five minutes silently listing the problem attributes on their individual work sheets. During the silent listing they do not speak to anyone else at their table.

At the end of five minutes, a staff member serving as a recorder moves to a large paper pad at each table. The recorder asks each client, one at a time, to give one problem from his or her work sheet. The recorder proceeds round-robin to receive an item from each client at the table in sequence, numbering each problem. He continues recording until all the problems group members choose to voice are listed.

After the clients have listed all their problems on the flip-board, the recorder leads the group in "serial discussion." Each problem on the pad, in the order listed, is discussed so that its meaning is clear to all participants. Reasons for agreement or disagreement are identified. New problems can also be added.

At the end of 20 or 30 minutes, the group is given 3" x 5" cards. Each client is asked to privately select (by number) the five problems he or she considers most crucial on the list. After selecting the priority problems, he is then asked to rank them. The recorder then collects the individual votes and records the votes of the group on each of the pad sheets. The extent of agreement is visually displayed by comparative rankings.

The group then discusses the anonymous rankings. Its task is to further clarify the items, not to create group pressure toward an artificial consensus. Unequal information or misunderstandings are resolved. The groups' final decision, however, is again arrived at by independent written rankings or ratings.

This technique, summarized in Figure 12–1, has successfully been utilized as a highly productive exploratory research tool. When combined with recorder notes elaborating on the clinical description of the priority problems based on client discussions, planners have a means of aggregating judgments between clients concerning the relative importance of various problems faced by single parents as represented by the groups on the client panel. They can also make comparisons between the individual groups.

Thus in 90 minutes, the planner is able to lead clients through the following six steps: (1) Silent Generation of Ideas in writing, (2) Round-Robin Recording of Ideas on a flip pad, (3) Serial Discussion for clarification, (4) Preliminary Vote on Problem Importance, (5) Discussion on the Preliminary Vote, and (6) Final Vote.

## UNDERLYING THEORETICAL BASES OF NGT

What is the underlying social-psychology involved in the NGT group process?

The NGT meeting just described combines into a sequential format group processes which facilitate (1) idea generation, (2) equal participation, and (3) judgmental aggregation.

Current research indicates that interaction actually inhibits

## Figure 12–1    Summary Leadership Guide for Conducting an NGT Meeting

Design Task
   Prepare the NGT Question.
      . Staff clarifies the Problem focus to which clients are to respond.
      . Print the NGT question on work sheets for each participant.

Preparing the Meeting Room
   Table Arrangement.
      . Tables arranged as an open "U" with a flip chart at the open end
        of the table.
      . Sufficient space between tables to avoid interference.
   Supplies.
      . Flip pad for each table and for the leader.
      . Nominal work sheets and pencils for each participant.
      . 3" x 5" cards (for ranking); or voting forms (for rating).
      . Felt pens.

Introducing the Meeting
   Welcoming Statement.
      . Cordial and warm welcome.
      . Statement of the importance of the task - to help planners understand
        the nature of the clients' contribution.
      . Statement of the use or purpose of the meeting's output.

Conduct the Nominal Group Process
Step 1.   Silent Generation of Ideas in Writing
   Process:
      . Present the problem identification question to the group in writing.
      . Verbally read the question.
      . Charge the group to write problem characteristics in brief phrases
        or statements.
      . Ask group members to work silently and independently.

Step 2.   Round-Robin Recording of Ideas on a Flip Pad.
   Process:
      . Record ideas as rapidly as possible.
      . Record ideas in the words used by group members.
      . Make the entire list visible by tearing off completed sheets and
        taping them with masking tape visible to all group members.

Step 3.   Serial Discussion for Clarification
   Process:
      . Verbally  define the purpose of the step.
        . To clarify the meaning of items
        . To explain reasons for agreement or disagreement
      . Indicate that final judgments will be expressed by voting so
        arguments are unnecessary.
      . Pace the group so that all ideas receive sufficient time
        for clarification.
      . Avoid forcing the member who originally lists the idea to be solely
        responsible for clarifying the item.

Step 4.   Preliminary Vote on Problem Importance.
   Process:
      . Ask each group to select from the entire list a specific number of
        priority (important) items.
      . Ask each group member to independently list his priority items on a
        sheet of paper or card.
      . Ask each group member to independently rank order or rate the selected
        priority items.
      . Hand in the votes, tally the votes, and record the results on the flip
        pad in front of the group.

**Figure 12–1    Continued**

```
Step 5.  Discussion of the Preliminary Vote.
   Process:
      . Define the role of the step as clarification, not pressure toward
        artificial consensus.
      . Keep the discussion brief.
      . Caution group members to think carefully about any changes they make
        in their voting.

Step 6.  Final Vote.
   Process:
      (Repeat Step Four)
```

idea generation. The benefits of Step One, Silent Listing, and Step Two, Round-Robin Recording, include adequate time for individual thinking and effort, avoidance of interruptions, avoidance of premature focusing on single ideas or problems, and increased problem centeredness. In effect, these steps maximize the ability of a client group to map all problem elements prior to attempts at clarification or ranking.

The structured interaction achieved by Step Two, Round-Robin Recording and Step Three, Serial Discussion, assures that all group members' ideas are noted and receive attention. These processes provide each group member time and opportunity to enter and clarify ideas. They eliminate dominance by aggressive personalities. The written record on the flip pad also helps the group to avoid losing ideas, thus increasing their ability to deal with a larger number of ideas.

The essential lesson from decision theory about aggregating judgments is that a group should follow a process of estimate-talk-estimate. Step Four, Preliminary Voting, allows estimates in the form of rankings or ratings which are recorded without identifying individuals. Step Five, Discussion of the Vote, helps the group to eliminate error due to unequal information or misunderstanding. Combined with Step Six, Final Voting, these three steps reduce social pressures, maximize group information, and avoid artificial consensus in coming to a decision about client problems.

Good summaries of the theory underlying NGT are available and indicated in the annotated bibliography. The point here is not to become distracted by the social and psychological dynamics of the NGT group meeting itself, since our central concern is with the value of such meetings in terms of needs assessment. Nonetheless, to put it in colloquial terms: "any" client panel or participation device "doesn't do it." NGT is a carefully constructed balance of individual thoughtfulness and idea generation, equalized information sharing, discussion for clarification, and mathematical aggregation of judgment. As such it is a particularly useful tool for clarifying the qualitative character of client problems.

## THE RELATIONSHIP OF NGT TO QUANTITATIVE TECHNIQUES

Clearly, even in terms of qualitative problem understanding, NGT is not a substitute for distributive data obtained from an appropriate sample. Qualitative assessments also require valid measurement. However, before quantifiable research measures dealing with qualitative or clinical concerns can be developed, the planner must possess: (1) a qualitative understanding of the problem as perceived by clients and (2) a knowledge of client jargon as opposed to professional symbolism to use in describing the problems. Otherwise the collected data may be invalid. NGT has often been used as an exploratory research tool to develop this qualitative problem understanding prior to the use of questionnaires or interview protocols when distributive data is essential to planning. In other instances, where distributive indicators are understood, NGT itself can be sufficient to generate the informed judgments and qualitative problem understanding required to proceed to subsequent planning phases: solution development and program design.

A qualitative understanding of client problems becomes more complex when multiple client and target groups are involved. In addition to its own language structure, each group may also have its own perspective concerning the attributes of the problem under investigation. Again NGT as a rapid and feasible pilot tool can help accentuate and decode the degree of client group differences.

## Summary

In summary, NGT can be used to effectively explore the qualitative nature of problems implicit in quantitative need assessments. It can:

1. Identify and enrich the researcher's understanding of problem attributes by providing judgmental problem identification, refined by priority ranking/ratings.
2. Focus attention on major areas of inquiry, defined by target groups in their own jargon, which may be pursued in greater detail by means of interview or questionnaire instruments.
3. Allow target groups to single out critical problems by means of a group process which is unthreatening and depersonalized.
4. Assist in the development of hypotheses and the formulation of questions for survey and interview field research.
5. Be implemented in a short time period for several different target groups at a low cost.

## Notes

1. Delbecq, A. L., Van de Ven, A. H., & Gustafson, H. *Group techniques for program planning: A guide to Nominal Group and Delphi processes.* Glenview, Ill: Scott-Foresman, 1975. A complete and explicit guide for professionals dealing with NGT and Delphi Processes, along with a theoretical summary and examples of applications.

2. Delbecq, A. L., & Van de Ven, A. H. Nominal versus interacting group processes for committee decision-making effectiveness. *Academy of Management Journal,* (January) 1971, *14*(1). The basic theoretical statement of social psychological theory underlying NGT.

3. Huber, G., & Delbecq, A. L. Guidelines for combining the judgments of individual group members in decision conferences. *Academy of Management Journal,* (June) 1972, *15*(2).

218 ASSESSING HEALTH AND HUMAN SERVICE NEEDS

4. Gustafson, D. H., Shukla, R. K., Delbecq, A. L., & Walster, G. W. A comparative study of differences in subjective likelihood estimates made by individuals, interacting groups, Delphi groups and Nominal Groups. *Organization Behavior and Human Performance*, 1973, *9*. Empirical studies of mathematical decision rules for aggregating group judgments.

5. Van de Ven, A., & Delbecq, A. L. The effectiveness of interacting, Delphi and Nominal Group decision making processes. *Academy of Management Journal*, (December) 1974, *17*(4).

Comparative evidence of group effectiveness.

Part IV

# NEED ASSESSMENT IN PROGRAM PLANNING

## INTRODUCTION

The purpose of need assessment is *not* to contribute to a general fund of knowledge. Need assessment is not basic research nor even, in the usual sense, applied research. It is a service activity that uses the tools of research for its own immediate specific ends. These ends can include systematic and ordered documentation of needs, program planning, and program change. Each chapter in this section deals with this service purpose of need assessment, recognizing the importance of identifying the program task and organizational environment.

Guttentag describes a systematic approach for selecting from among alternative program goals, including both values and information from a variety of sources. This yields "utilities" for different alternatives that serve to quantify service goals. Sundel describes the steps involved in his conducting a need assessment in a live, dynamic service agency and the requirements that organizational conditions and service considerations place on the need assessor. Murrell conceptualizes the process of converting need assessment information into service utilization and suggests eight steps that would facilitate such usage. Demone draws on his long experience as a planner to illustrate the complexities of using data for service decisions and identifies the conditions under which one should and should *not* attempt a need assessment.

Apparent in all of these chapters is a recognition of the importance of the political arena and the need to coordinate the activities of need assessors and data users. Otherwise, as has too often happened in the past, the mismatch between need assessment and service agency ideologies can lead to misuse and even nonutilization of assessment data.

*Chapter 13*

# THE INTEGRATION OF NEED ASSESSMENT INTO EVALUATION

*Marcia Guttentag*

In order to present the topic of need assessment in the context of an overall evaluation plan, this chapter will (1) briefly review some of the evaluation requirements of Community Mental Health Center (CMHC) legislation other than need assessment; (2) enumerate some of the key issues in need assessment; (3) present an overall evaluation paradigm, which makes it possible to integrate need assessment into other evaluation requirements; and (4) draw conclusions about the place of need assessment in evaluation. Need assessment is only one of a number of evaluation requirements in the CMHC evaluation regulations. Additional requirements are recommended as standards for CMHC evaluation. Data must be collected, analyzed, and evaluated on the following topics:

1. Causes—as related to both services and outcome.
2. Availability, accessibility, and acceptability of services.
3. The match between services rendered and demographic attributes of the catchment area.
4. Impact of services on the community, such as on hospitalization rates, suicide, etc.

With only a mandatory 2 percent of operating funds for evaluation, a large number of other evaluation requirements must be considered in addition to need assessment.[1] Effectiveness in meeting the needs of residents of the catchment area must be assessed. This will entail both measurement of patient outcome as well as program goals, developed on the basis of need assessment and action steps to meet the needs. Actually it seems to imply a management-by-objective approach in some form at least. Goal formulation will be stressed as a basis for evaluation. Quality of services will need to be measured through utilization and peer review process. Citizens from the catchment area must participate in both the planning and evaluation of services.

These specifications in the administrative regulations require that need assessment be open to some type of peer review and citizen participation and that need assessment be integrated into overall programmatic goals for a health service program. How can one therefore integrate need assessment measures with both peer review systems and an overall evaluation paradigm? Even more important, how shall decisions be made about what needs are to be assessed, and how shall measures of need assessment be related to overall programmatic goals? In the comments that follow, an overall evaluation paradigm is offered for use in health services fields that can integrate need assessment with overall programmatic goals. The paradigm is a decision-theoretic multiattribute utility approach combined with Bayesian statistics, affectionately known as the MAUT-Bayesian approach to planning and evaluation.

## PEER REVIEW AS AN ESSENTIAL PART OF CMHC EVALUATION

Accountability has become a key issue in health services. But, accountable to whom? Because health services are, by their very nature, community based and oriented programs, many have from the start realized that citizen representation in catchment areas is a necessary part of the peer review process. Health service planners have discussed the importance of peer review in both the planning and evaluation of health services from the very initiation of programs. Where does need assessment fit? What conceptual frameworks and what methodologies can be used to build in the peer review process and citizen participation as an integral part of planning and evaluation? And, how can measures of need assessment be used in such planning and evaluation?

The answer, I think, is that a usable evaluation paradigm must separate the specification of the goals of a health program from the technical planning and evaluation of programs. Such a paradigm should permit citizens to indicate what their values and overall goals are for health programs. Professionals then can formulate the content of services that they believe will meet these objectives. Evaluation is the determination of the extent to which these citizen-generated goals are being met. Need assessment measures can then be used in both the planning and evaluation of health service programs.

As Warheit, Bell, and Schwab[2] have so aptly put it:

> Mental health needs assessment studies permit community mental health centers to do the following: (1) to identify the types and extent of mental health needs present in the community being served; (2) to secure data which will permit centers to evaluate systematically their existing programs in terms of the identified needs; (3) to alter existing programs and/or to structure new ones in keeping with the community's needs and care patterns; and, (4) to develop a sound baseline of research data on which later evaluation, outcome and impact studies can be conducted.

But if these aims are to be realized for the full integration of need assessment studies with planning and evaluation, then the overall evaluation paradigm for health services must have certain additional characteristics. These other characteristics must include:

1. *Multiple measurement of goals and of outcomes.* Since the goals of any health program are always complex and multiple, a useful evaluation paradigm must have multiple measurement requirements built into it, not added at the discretion of the researcher.

2. *Data inclusiveness.* All forms of measurement are expensive. It is therefore essential that in health evaluation,

no data be thrown out or omitted because it does not meet the exacting standards of classical statistical tests. A useful evaluation paradigm for health programs should be data inclusive, that is, observational data, formal measurement, archival data, etc., should all be used when they are available. Further, the evaluation paradigm should permit the integration of widely varying types of data. The different measures of need assessment, for example, should be able to be integrated by the statistical system that is used in the evaluation.

3. *Values and goals.* A peer review should generate measures of desired program outcomes so that progress toward these goals may be evaluated.

4. *Continuous feedback.* Continuous or intermittent feedback should be an integral part of the evaluation paradigm. Relevant data on need assessment and on program effectiveness should be available *whenever* decisions must be made.

## THE MAUT-BAYESIAN PARADIGM

The MAUT-Bayesian paradigm, a decision-theoretic multiattribute utility and Bayesian statistical evaluation paradigm, meets the characteristics and criteria that have been enumerated. This version is one from a family of multiattribute, decision-theoretic approaches. It is oriented toward easy communication and use in environments in which time is short and decision makers are multiple. It is a method that is psychologically meaningful to decision makers. The judgments they are required to give are intuitively reasonable.

The essence of any multiattribute utility measurement is that each outcome to be evaluated is located on each dimension of value by a procedure that may consist of experimentation, naturalistic observation, judgment, or some combination of these. We call these "location measures," and they are combined by means of an aggregation rule, most often simply a weighted linear

combination. The weights are numbers describing the importance of each dimension of value relative to the others. These
numbers are judgmentally obtained.

The building of the planning and evaluation model consists
of ten steps that result in a simple matrix. The matrix is the
structure within which plans are presented, and it is revised at
every step of the evaluation. Most abstractly, the steps are as
follows:[3]

*Step 1:* Identify the person or organization whose utilities
are to be maximized. If, as is often the case, several
organizations have stakes and voices in the decision, they must all be identified. People who can
speak for them must be identified and induced to
cooperate. That is the beginning of the implementation of the peer review process required for
much health program evaluation.

*Step 2:* Identify the issue or issues (i.e., decisions) to which
the utilities needed are relevant. The same health
programs may have many different values, depending on context and purpose. In general, utility is a function of the evaluator, the entity being
evaluated, and the purpose for which the evaluation is being made.

*Step 3:* Identify the programs to be evaluated. This includes not only all current programs, but any con-
ceivable action alternatives, tried or untried.

*Step 4:* Identify the relevant dimensions of value. It is
important not to be too expansive at this stage.
The number of relevant dimensions of value
should be kept down, for reasons that will be apparent shortly. This can often be done by restating
and combining goals or by moving upward in a
goal hierarchy, thereby using fewer, more general
values. Even more important, it can be done by
simply omitting the less important goals. There is
no requirement that the list evolved in this step be
complete, and much reason to hope that it won't

be.Pragmatically, these values can be elicited from peer review groups under consensus rules or from individuals privately.

*Step 5:* Rank the dimensions in order of importance. This ranking job, like Step 4, can be performed by an individual, by representatives of conflicting values, groups acting separately, or by those representatives acting as a group. Our preferred technique is to try group process first, mostly to get the arguments on the table and to make it more likely that the participants start from a common information base, and then to get separate judgments from each individual. The separate judgments will differ, of course, both here and in the following step.

*Step 6:* Rate dimensions in importance, preserving ratios. To do this, start by assigning the least important dimension an importance of 10. (We use 10 rather than 1 to permit subsequent judgments to be finely graded and nevertheless made in integers.) Now consider the next-least-important dimension. How many times more important (if any) is it than the least important? Assign it a number that reflects that ratio. Continue on up the list checking each set of implied ratios as each new judgment is made. Thus, if a dimension is assigned a weight of 20, while another is assigned a weight of 80, it means that the 20 dimension is ¼ as important as the 80 dimension. And so on. By the time you get the most important dimensions, there will be many checks to perform; typically, respondents will want to revise previous judgments to make them consistent with present ones. That's fine; they can do so. Once again, individual differences are likely to arise.

*Step 7:* Sum the importance weights, divide each by the sum, and multiply by 100. This is a purely computational step which converts importance weights into numbers that, mathematically, are rather like probabilities. The choice of a 0-to-100 scale is, of course, purely arbitrary.

At this step the folly of including too many dimensions at Step 4 becomes glaringly apparent. If 100 points are to be distributed over a set of dimensions, and some dimensions are very much more important than others, then the less important dimensions will have nontrivial weights only if there are not too many of them. As a rule of thumb, eight dimensions is plenty, and 15 is too many. Knowing this, you will want, at Step 4, to discourage respondents from being too finely analytical; rather gross dimensions will be just right. Moreover, it may occur that the list of dimensions will be revised later and that revision, if it occurs, will typically consist of including more rather than fewer.

*Step 8:* Measure the location of each entity being evaluated on each dimension. The word *measure* is used rather loosely here. There are three classes of dimensions: purely subjective, partly subjective, and purely objective. The purely subjective dimensions are perhaps the easiest; you simply get an appropriate expert to estimate the position of that entity on that dimension on a 0-to-100 scale, where 0 is defined as the minimum plausible value on that dimension and 100 is defined as the maximum plausible value.

A partly subjective dimension is one in which the units of measurement are objective, but the locations of the entities must be subjectively estimated.

A wholly objective dimension is one that can be measured rather objectively, in objective units, before the decision.

The final task in Step 8 is to convert measures from the partly subjective and wholly objective dimensions into the 0-to-100 scale in which 0 is minimum plausible and 100 is maximum plausible.

It may be useful to conceptualize this step as the creation of a matrix. The importance-weighted values head each of the columns, and the programs, or action alternatives, are the rows. Each of the cells in the matrix, in Step 8, receives a "location measure." On a subjective scale of 0–100, how likely is it, given what you know now, that this program (or action alternative) will maximize this value?

Such a matrix might look like this (Figure 13–1)

Step 9:  Calculate utilities for entities. The equation is $U_i = {}_iw_ju_ij$, remembering that ${}_jwj = 100$. $U_i$ is the aggregate utility for the ith entity. $w_j$ is the normalized importance weight of the jth dimension of value, and $u_{ij}$ is the rescaled position of the ith entity of the jth dimension. Thus $w_j$ is the output of Step 7,

## Matrix

| | Importance Weighted Values | | | | | |
| | A 20.1 | B 11.2 | C 7.9 | E | F | D |
|---|---|---|---|---|---|---|
| Program 1 | | | | | | |
| Program 2 | | | | | | |
| Program 3 | | | | | | |
| Program 4 | | | | | | |
| Program 5 | | | | | | |
| Program 6 | | | | | | |

(Health Programs or Alternatives)

Figure 13–1

and $u_{ij}$ is the output of Step 8. The equation, of course, is nothing more than the formula for a weighted average.

*Step 10:*  Decide. If a single act is to be chosen, the rule is simple: maximize $U_i$. If a subset of $i$ is to be chosen, then the subset for which $_iU_i$ is maximum is best.

Costs are nearly always one of the value dimensions.

## INTERPERSONAL AND INTERGROUP DISAGREEMENTS

Nothing in the preceding discussion ensures that different respondents will come up with similar numbers, and such agreements are indeed rare. Although multiattribute utility measurement procedures can be expected to reduce the magnitude of disagreements, they cannot and should not eliminate them. What then?

There are two kinds of disagreements. Disagreements at Step 8 are like disagreements among different thermometers measuring the same temperature. If they are not too large, an average can be taken. If they are, then we are likely to suspect that some of the thermometers are not working properly and to discard their readings. In general, judgmentally determined "location measures" should reflect expertise, and typically, different value dimensions require different kinds of expertise and therefore different experts. In some practical contexts, the problem of disagreement at Step 8 can be avoided entirely by the simple expedient of asking only the best available expert for each dimension to make judgments about that dimension, or of using the best available data.

Disagreements at steps 5 and 6 are another matter. These are the essence of conflicting values, and they should be respected as much as possible. There is no reason why each of the different participating groups in the planning process should not have their own separate matrix. In practice, we frequently do just that.

Groups can adopt various decision rules, for example, in the weighted-averaging spirit of multiattribute utility measurement, by assigning a weight to each of the disagreeing parties and then calculating weighted-average importance weights.

If there is no decision rule to resolve disagreement, the evaluation is carried on separately for each of the disagreeing individuals or groups. Thus the same data can lead citizen groups with different values to come to different conclusions. The familiar political processes, by means of which society functions in spite of conflicting interests, come into play. The evaluation simply provides accurate information to the competing groups.

## Need Assessment Integrated into the Overall Evaluation Paradigm

Let us now return to some of the issues that were raised earlier in this paper about the ways in which the assessment must be integrated into an overall evaluation paradigm. It may perhaps be clearest to illustrate the ways in which need assessment can be integrated by using a concrete illustration.

Let us suppose that in filling in the MAUT-Bayesian matrix that the program alternatives include in-patient services, partial-hospitalization, after-care, consultation in education, children services, alcoholism and substance abuse programs, and transitional care programs. If we then fill in the decision-theoretic matrix, these would be the actual programs being evaluated (see Figure 13–2).

For the sake of this illustration, let us also suppose that we have gone through the MAUT process with program decision

**MAUT - Bayesian Matrix**

| Health Program Alternatives | A | B | C | D | E | F |
|---|---|---|---|---|---|---|
| | 10.85 | 10.85 | 9.04 | | | |
| Inpatient services | 84 | 34 | 23 | | | |
| Partial - hospitalization | 26 | 13 | 24 | | | |
| Aftercare | 48 | 81 | 34 | | | |
| Consultation in education | 12 | 32 | 35 | | | |
| Children services | 31 | 22 | 33 | | | |
| Alcoholism & substance abuse | 67 | 64 | 21 | | | |
| Transitional care | 34 | 34 | 12 | | | |

Figure 13–2 MAUT-Bayesian Matrix

makers and we know that the following are a few of their most important values:

    A.   Institutional survival, programs that are popular with the community and funding agencies (importance weight: 10.85)

    B.   Meeting the needs of disadvantaged groups in the community (importance weight: 10.85)

    C.   Families' options in the community are strengthened (importance weight: 9.04). Of course there may be a great many more important values.

Let us presume that during the planning process the experts had some data already available which related each of these programs to three values. Therefore, we see in each cell a prior probability.

Now let us turn to the way in which need assessment evaluation plans can be made. Let us presume that there is a choice between field surveys, which are an expensive type of need assessment, or the use of the nominal group method[4] and/or the use of the mental health demographic profile system and the key informant method. Given the nature of the three most important values, it would appear that vis-a-vis value A, need assessment data would not be relevant. For values B and C, need assessment data would certainly be relevant. However, if there are prior probabilities based on the knowledge of experts, and there are also a great many other values for which data is relevant, it would seem likely that a method like the nominal group method or the key informant method combined with some type of social indicators method would be used. These would permit the revision of the prior probabilities in each cell to posterior probabilities given this type of needs assessment data. Further, the use of these need assessment measures would make it possible to revise decisions continuously, in time for what decision makers and program people both need.

Note that by using the MAUT-Bayesian approach to planning in evaluation, one can take advantage of what decision makers already know. After all, we all know that there is no substitute for going out to the field and seeing what programs are doing and who is being served. Further, in a great many health programs, people who are knowledgeable about the community already know a great deal about the nature of the needs in that community. This paradigm presumes that there may be information already known to decision makers. Note that this is not the way in which basic research is conducted by social scientists. In basic research, which is conducted according to classical methods, the assumption is that once an hypothesis has been derived on the basis of theory and past research, one knows nothing about whether the hypothesis is likely to be true. That is the very basis of null hypothesis testing. Thus the MAUT-Bayesian paradigm requires a style of thinking that is different from the way in which social scientists have usually been taught to think about laboratory experimentation. However, the reason that this paradigm is so appropriate for evaluation is that it does make use of all the sources of data, both past and present, that can be relevant to decision making. Thus, it is both data inclusive and based on multiple measurement. The Bayesian system itself makes it possible to integrate data from a wide variety of data sources. Thus, using this approach, all sources of data can be used to help revise decisions. Thus, data on need assessment based on field surveys, on social indicators, on key informants, on nominal group methods, and a whole variety of other methodologies can be integrated to revise differences successively. Further, using the overall Bayesian framework makes it possible to make decisions about how much of the resources should go into the various methods for obtaining need assessment data.

## CONCLUSION

The MAUT-Bayesian evaluation system makes possible the use of what is already known about the needs of the various populations served by any health service program. And, it uses much that can be inferred without additional need assessment measurement.

## NOTES

1.  Davis, H. Personal communication from Dr. Howard Davis, National Institute of Mental Health, Rockville, Maryland.

2.  Warheit, G. J., Bell, R. A., & Schwab, J. J. *Planning for change: Needs assessment approaches*. National Institute of Mental Health Publication. Washington, D.C. United States Government Printing Office, August 1975.

3.  Edwards, W., Guttentag, M., & Snapper, K. A decision-theoretic approach to evaluation research. In E. Struening & M. Guttentag (Eds.), *Handbook of Evaluation Research* (Vol. 1) Beverly Hills, Calif.: Sage Publications, 1975.

4.  Delbecq, A. *Nominal Group Method*. Paper presented at the First National Conference on Need Assessment, Louisville, Kentucky, 1976.

*Chapter 14*

# CONDUCTING NEED ASSESSMENT IN A COMMUNITY MENTAL HEALTH CENTER

*Martin Sundel*

Community mental health centers have become increasingly sensitive to pressures from both sponsors and citizenry that their programs be responsive to community needs. The Community Mental Health Centers Ammendments of 1975[1] require, among other things, that a mental health center commit 2 percent of its annual operating expenses for ongoing program evaluation.[2] The National Health Planning and Resources Development Act of 1974[3] requires that national health planning goals based on the priorities of population needs be developed and that such goals be described, wherever feasible, in quantitative terms. This legislation also calls for the establishment of health systems agencies that will assemble and analyze health data about the residents in their geographic service areas.

The application of need assessment technology provides a baseline for evaluating community mental health programs. If mental health services are planned and implemented with the intention of determining their community impact, epidemiologic data should be obtained for a wide range of conditions and problems related to emotional and mental disorders.

This chapter describes the approach taken by a large community mental health program in establishing and implementing need assessment studies relevant for program planning and evaluation, and for contributing empirical knowledge related to assessment of community needs. The strategy used in developing intra- and interorganizational conditions conducive for implementation of a comprehensive community survey will be discussed.

River Region Mental Health-Mental Retardation Board (renamed Seven County Services, Inc. in 1978) is one of fifteen regional mental health programs in Kentucky. It is mandated to serve a population of approximately 800,000 people in a seven-county area in northcentral Kentucky, including Louisville, the largest city in the state.

In addition to four comprehensive mental health centers, River Region operates an alcohol and drug treatment facility and also manages, or has affiliations with, other special units including partial hospitalization and aftercare programs, mental retardation group homes and intermediate care facilities, and drug and alcohol abuse programs.

The sociodemographic characteristics of the communities served by River Region are extremely heterogeneous, including rural, suburban, and urban populations with varying levels of income and diverse ethnic backgrounds. Median family incomes in 1970 for census tract populations in River Region ranged from $2,783 to $32,676 per year. The annual median income for all families in Jefferson County, which includes the city of Louisville, was $7,875. The percentage of black residents, ranging from 0 to 99.7 across census tracts, was approximately 15 percent in Jefferson County.

In August 1972, I moved from Boston to Louisville and established the Research and Evaluation Department at River Region Mental Health-Mental Retardation (MH-MR) Board. When I arrived in Louisville, two catchment areas (A and D) were operational, while another two (B and C) were newly-funded and organizing for implementation of service programs. Catchment Areas A and D each had one mental health center, along with several satellite operations in church and community buildings. The September 1972 reorganization plan established four comprehensive service centers in each of the four areas. As a result, the regional progam included some service centers that had been in operation for several years and others that were at the stage of seeking staff and planning services. In conceptualizing the evaluation program, an attempt was made to assess the rapidly evolving programs according to their stages of development. The evaluation model presented by Tripodi, Fellin, and Epstein[4] provided a basis for operationalizing evaluation issues in relation to program development at initiation, contact, or implementation stage.

Staff patterns were continually changing during the first half year of my job. The number of staff doubled from 150 to over 300 persons in the first six months and continued to increase dramatically, reaching 700 by December 1973. Accordingly, River Region's budget grew from eight million to over ten million dollars. In July 1974, River Region took over the operation of a state hospital which added over 500 employees and raised the overall budget to 16 million dollars.

One of my first steps in formulating a need assessment program was to visit each center and meet with the staff to learn more about their ability to describe their surrounding communities; many of them had little but impressionistic knowledge. Area D had the oldest mental health center, established in 1969, and the consultation and education staff had considerable knowledge of their environment. These staff were actively addressing salient mental health issues by participating in local community planning groups and were familiar with their clients' neighborhoods. Staff in the newer centers were also beginning to develop knowledge of their communities. Some center staff were already attempting to compare client data with census and community data. In several centers, staff placed multicolored pins in maps to locate clients in neighborhoods and streets where they lived. The colored pins represented geographic groupings of client problems or characteristics.

The multicolored pin method provided information showing how different environments were related to clients coming to the mental health center for help. A drug program manager was shown how to locate neighborhoods and streets where heroin addiction and other drug problems occurred with highest prevalence by pinpointing the addresses of River Region clients with these problems. This approach was also used to help drug program staff systematically focus their community outreach and education activities.

I made frequent appointments at the various centers to present information regarding program evaluation, epidemiology of mental disorders, and need assessment. These interchanges with staff resulted in greater familiarity with important issues related to their communities. I quickly found that need assessment was a far less sensitive topic than was evaluation of service effectiveness. Relationships that developed with staff around need assessment activities, however, often provided the basis for increased program evaluation efforts.

Systematic knowledge of community needs and resources was an important requirement for providing baseline data that could be utilized in evaluating the impact of River Region services. A systematic approach to need assessment and program evaluation in the centers required a uniform regional framework; therefore, a strategy was designed for assessing community needs and resources that would be integrally related to the total organization's evaluation program.[5] The assessment was to be based on a variety of environmental data including census statistics, surveys, media reports, and other agency statistics. In addition, the program would include key informant and rates-under-treatment studies.[6] A standardized format was developed for presenting and sharing relevant census and community data with service center staff. According to the plan, assessment data relevant for each of the centers would be provided; the service center data could be combined to provide demographic profiles for each of the four areas.

The initial strategy called for compilation of a Community Assessment Profile (CAP) for each of the centers. The social area analysis format suggested by Goldsmith and Unger[7] provided a model for structuring the profile outline. When completed, the Community Assessment Profile included 62 items classified into the following five categories: (1) population characteristics (including ethnicity, age, and sex); (2) family/nonfamily characteristics (including household size, family composition, and family life cycle); (3) social characteristics (including education and job status); (4) economic characteristics (including employment, family income, and persons and families below poverty level); and (5) housing characteristics (including items related to owner- and renter-occupied units, mobility, and crowding conditions). Data from surveys conducted by other community organizations, as well as by center staff, furnished additional descriptive information. A more detailed presentation of this approach has been reported elsewhere.[8]

Many of the 1973 CAP items were based on those covered in the Mental Health Demographic Profile System (MHDPS) that was being developed by the National Institute of Mental Health (NIMH). Thus, comparisons of data for each census tract could be made with NIMH statistics for catchment area, county, state, and nation.[9–11] A system was also devised for collecting client data that could be compared with the CAP data. In this way, the characteristics of River Region clients could be compared with those of the total population.[8] In order for research staff to compare client and census data, it was essential for center staff to accurately record client information on the application and intake forms. Center staff became more involved in collecting client demographic data after they had experienced the utility of comparing client data with that of residents in the center's geographic area.

Research staff met with the consultation and education staff of each center to assist in interpreting the profiles and relating the data to particular issues and problems experienced by the center. Center staff became more aware of accessibility problems for clients who appeared to be underserved in proportion to their numbers in the census tract population. In addition, center supervisors were involved in analyzing the data and drawing implications for community outreach and center planning.

This need assessment program generally increased center staff's knowledge of their communities and assisted in setting consultation and education priorities. When program and facility standards were developed for River Region in the fall of 1973, specific items were included in the evaluation standards that related to determining and rating a center's involvement in community assessment and program evaluation activities.[12] In order to obtain a satisfactory rating on the community assessment standards, center staff were required to furnish evidence of their activities in this area. In accordance with these standards, the consultation and education staff began to formulate objectives that specifically mention need assessment activities and criteria for achievement.

In 1973–1974, a mass media preventive education program entitled "Alternatives" was carried out by River Region MH-MR Board. A survey was conducted to determine community awareness of mental health services. Mental health attitudes related to messages broadcast on radio and television were also measured using a pretest-posttest time series design. The survey provided information showing the impact of River Region on community awareness of mental health services.[13]

These preliminary efforts in establishing a community need assessment program helped a rapidly growing organization become more knowledgeable about its environment. For example, the CAP profile could be compared with client data to determine the extent to which a center was serving clients with certain characteristics. If individuals 65 and over represented 3 percent of a center's client population while they formed 26 percent of community residents, this could indicate that center services were inaccessible to or inadequate for such clients. Of course, center staff would also have to consider the existence of other community resources as a possible explanation for any such discrepancy between the number of elderly clients and the actual size of the elderly population. Systems such as CAP and MHDPS could thus be of considerable practical utility for human service organizations and their sponsors concerned with providing adequate services to client groups that are frequently underserved.[14]

It became apparent, however, that in order to measure the extent to which prevention goals were being accomplished, a more comprehensive epidemiologic approach was required. Psychosocial and health statuses of community residents could only by hypothesized on the basis of data such as the CAP profile. A divergence of service utilization rates from subpopulation proportions might not indicate service deficiencies, for example, if the psychosocial and health statuses of a particular group were satisfactory or better. Thus, determination of service deficiencies for a community required a reasonably accurate assessment of the psychosocial and health statuses of the general population.

While various methods have been used to identify community needs,[6] the survey has been useful for determining the distribution of mental and emotional disorders in the population.[15–23]

In the fall of 1974, several factors created an optimal climate for conducting a comprehensive needs assessment survey. River Region MH-MR Board[24] had arrived at a fairly stable funding position, and the rapid acceleration of services and program development had reached an asymptote. A Goal-Oriented Record Keeping (GORK) System[25] was implemented throughout River Region to provide a systematic framework for evaulating services. The Survey of Mental Health Needs in Kentucky,[26] sponsored by the Kentucky Association for Mental Health and the Kentucky Psychiatric Association, had recommended that epidemiologic research be focused on factors related to the occurrence of mental and emotional disorders within the community. Drs. John Schwab and Roger Bell of the University of Louisville Department of Psychiatry had expressed an interest in conducting a survey of the Louisville metropolitan area in collaboration with River Region's research staff.

Before a survey could be undertaken, sanctions and funding were required from the River Region administration. This process involved negotiation of mutually satisfactory arrangements between River Region and the Department of Psychiatry. One question raised frequently by the administrators was whether or not mental health needs could actually be measured. This question aroused considerable discussion, especially in relation to defining mental health.[27,28] Several administrators and clinicians were concerned that the concept of mental health was too broad or nebulous to be operationalized and quantified. Analysis and discussion of appropriate methodologies for identifying and assessing mental health needs, as well as previous work carried out in this area, led to an interest by the River Region administration in conducting a comprehensive survey. A procedure was established for the submission and review of a research proposal. If the proposal were approved, funds for the survey would be allocated from internal monies.

The implementation of a community need assessment survey requires considerable attention to aligning organizational conditions conducive to conceptualization, planning, funding, and coordinating a large-scale project. As Director of the Research Department, it was necessary for me to establish the priority of the need assessment in relation to other research efforts. The rationale for the project was carefully explained to the Executive Director and other program and administrative staff in order to enlist their support and make them aware of the benefits that could accrue to the organization. It was essential that appropriate expertise be available in designing and implementing the survey to justify the organization's expense, as well as to ascertain the soundness of the scientific design of the study. Almost a year-and-a-half before the project was initiated, negotiations were held with the Chairman of the Department of Psychiatry and his staff regarding the proposed collaborative study.

In October 1974, a proposal was submitted to the Executive Director. The objectives of the project were stated as (1) identifying the social, physical, and mental health needs of each catchment area and (2) developing an approach to comprehensive need assessment that could serve as a model for other catchment areas in Kentucky, as well as other states. According to the proposal, over 1,300 randomly selected households would be interviewed to determine: (1) existing family needs and (2) ways in which the families were meeting their needs from formal and informal community resources and caregivers. This initial proposal set forth the respective responsibilities and roles of Department of Psychiatry and River Region staff in conceptualizing, operationalizing, and implementing the survey. Because of fiscal and organizational problems, final approval took another year.

The survey would provide a number of benefits for River Region and the community. It was designed so that follow-up surveys at various intervals could determine the impact of mental health services on the prevalence of mental and emotional disorders. If a severe untreated mental health problem was discovered, the individual or family could be referred to River Region or other community caregivers. It was expected that, by participating in the survey, individuals and families would become aware of River Region and other community services and they could thereby function as informal referral agents in their community. Impediments to receiving care could be identified so that agencies could take these into account in program planning and operations. The project would augment the scientific approach to need assessment and would enhance the findings of other studies related to community mental health needs and attitudes. Finally, the data could help individuals in key policy-making roles at state and local levels establish priorities. Conceptualization of the model to be applied in constructing the interview schedule had begun in the summer of 1974. A variety of need assessment instruments and relevant literature were gathered and reviewed. It was intended that the survey would generate useful data on the community, rather than merely replicating other studies. For this reason, it was important to obtain input for the survey items from a variety of individuals within and without River Region. Specific concerns of River Region and the community that had to be taken into account in developing this instrument included a tornado that the Louisville area experienced in April 1974, the Alternatives mass media and preventive education project, and recently instituted court-ordered school busing.

After considerable discussion, a 498-item interview schedule was developed. The instrument contained items in the following areas: (1) basic social and demographic characteristics of families; (2) interpersonal and familial networks; (3) a comprehensive medical systems screen; (4) life satisfactions/aspirations; (5) a stressful life events inventory; (6) a comprehensive psychiatric rating scale; (7) natural disasters and community crises; (8) family interactional patterns denoting difficulties as well as assets in family life; (9) utilization of formal and informal support systems; (10) an assertiveness scale based on behavioral concepts[29]; and (11) attitudes toward and utilization of health, mental health, and social services. The project was entitled The Louisville Metropolitan Health and Family Life Studies, a name that was intended to provide a broader community base of support than designation of sponsorship by any one agency. I was named project director, and I hired a staff person to coordinate and supervise the interviewers.

Various community agencies were informed about the project prior to its implementation. Discussions were held with staff from a Human Service Coordinating Agency to explore possibilities for collaboration since this group was planning to conduct a need assessment for the elderly population. Meetings were held with staff from the Regional Health Planning Agency to enlist their support for the project and to discuss areas in which the project could be helpful to them. Planning organizations in Louisville were becoming increasingly aware of the implications of the National Health Planning and Resources Development Act,[3] since staff from those agencies might be selected to play a role in administering the projected health systems agency responsible for the geographic region including Louisville.

In the middle of November 1975, the survey was initiated with interviews of individuals in 300 households selected through sampling of six different census tracts. These six tracts were selected on the basis of a recent social indicators study conducted by George Warheit, Roger Bell, Charles Holzer, Lynn Robbins, and their colleagues in Florida and Kentucky. The study was designed to examine the differences in quality of life among the various census tracts in the River Region area and to triangulate with the need assessment data collected by the Louisville study, as well as provide data for comparison with Florida studies. The indicators included socioeconomic rank, housing rank, crime rank, health rank, and pollution rank. A weighted average of ranks on component indices was calculated and used to determine the 10 best and 10 worst census tracts in the River Region area. The six census tracts used in the initial survey were selected from these 20.

After the initial survey was completed, the sampling scheme was developed for the major survey. After enumerating 253,000 households in the seven county area, a statistical probability sample of 2,500 (1 percent) potential respondents was drawn. Later comparisons with census data were planned to determine the sample's representativeness.

A multistage probability sampling design was employed using the Kish[30] method of randomizing respondents within households. All respondents in each household aged 18 years and older were listed by sex and age on the household face sheet. Sheets were precoded to indicate which individual in the household was to be selected as the respondent.

The interview schedule was administered in the home of each respondent. The interviewers also gave copies of two instruments for assessing child mental health needs to respondents after the interview was completed.

In undertaking our comprehensive survey, considerable attention was given to recruitment of interviewers. We found that in order to retain interested and competent interviewers, proper training, supervision, and feedback had to be provided. In addition, continuous support on both the information and socioemotional levels had to be given to maintain the interviewers' motivation and interest. A weekly meeting held with the interviewers involved discussion and analysis of their problems along with suggestions for realistic solutions or ways of coping. Group problem-solving seemed to help interviewers cope with the considerable frustration generated by the interviewing process and maintain a more objective perspective on their work. An interviewer coordinator who would take the time to discuss problems, situations, and solutions experienced by interviewers could contribute a great deal to maintaining their morale and effectiveness.

Community mental health centers must be concerned realistically about the logistics and cost of conducting a comprehensive survey. Before undertaking the project, researchers and administrators should calculate the costs involved in developing instrumentation—validating its content and reproducing it; drawing the sample; conducting the interviews; processing and analyzing data; and hiring, training, and maintaining competent interviewers. River Region's commitment of resources did not come immediately, and our patience and persistence were required in establishing the various resources and costs involved and explaining their necessity to the administration. It was especially important to be patient during the periods of fiscal uncertainty in the organization while maintaining the viability of the proposal. After resources were committed to the needs assessment survey, the project was established as a priority for River Region, despite fiscal cutbacks. The implementation of the project involved a substantial increase in the number and range of contacts and interchanges between the research department and other River Region departments. These interactions created greater visibility for the activities of the research department and its use of agency resources.

A number of conclusions drawn from our experience might prove helpful to other organizations.

1.  The purposes of the project should be clearly thought through in terms of the type of information needed by the organization and the community, as well as that desired for contributing scientific knowledge.
2.  Organizational resources for conducting a survey should be assessed, especially in terms of the available research capabilities.
3.  Opportunities to collaborate with other organizations where expertise is available, such as university departments, should be explored.
4.  Negotiations with other organizations should be explicit in terms of responsibilities and roles in the project.
5.  It is advantageous for the Project Director to be an agency staff person with direct access and responsibility to the Executive Director.
6.  Input for survey items and objectives for the study should be drawn from agency staff, board members, community issues and concerns, and previous research findings.
7.  A mechanism should be established for gaining sanctions from major planning groups and community agencies. The local Better Business Bureau, police department, and other community sources should be informed that project staff will be interviewing community residents.
8.  Project expenses should be monitored through a systematic accounting procedure.
9.  Written reports and oral presentations should be provided regularly to keep the Executive Director, Board, agency staff, and other sponsors informed.
10. Mechanisms for dissemination of findings should include collaboration with relevant community planning groups, as well as with key agency staff.

It is particularly timely for community mental health centers to become actively engaged in assessing community needs. In December 1975, the Division of Community Mental Health Centers[1] issued a working draft of principles for the accreditation of community mental health services programs. The draft was submitted for review under a contract for the development of

standards for community mental health centers supported by
NIMH and related Federal agencies. The principles for the standards related to need assessment included the following:[31]

> The program shall establish baseline data depicting the
> geographic, demographic, cultural, and socioeconomic fea-
> tures of the service area. The program shall establish base-
> line data for target populations within the services area. The
> program shall maintain biological, psychological, social and
> cultural profiles on consumers in the service area. These
> profiles should be organized by functional area and activity
> to assist clinical management staff. These profiles shall pro-
> tect individual consumer identification. The program shall
> provide for cross-sectional and longitudinal analysis of ser-
> vices and need patterns.
>
> These principles, if adopted, can provide guidance to
> community mental health centers in developing their needs
> assessment programs, especially if funds are made contin-
> gent upon substantive efforts in this area.

Community mental health centers will become increasingly
involved in planning efforts to address the needs of specialized
populations. In October 1977, the NIMH funded a series of 20
community support program (CSP) contracts with state governments across the country.[32] The purpose of these demonstration
projects was to stimulate development of community-based care
and services to meet the needs of chronic, seriously emotionally
disabled adults living outside of institutions. Each project was
required to submit to NIMH a need assessment report including
data on the number, location, demographics, and service needs
of the target population. These data were to be used in formulating a statewide action plan for developing community support
systems.

The President's Commission on Mental Health has called for
the establishment of a nationwide program of performance contracts with state mental health agencies to improve the care of the
chronically, mentally ill.[33] Implementation plans for this program will probably build on experience from CSP demonstration
projects. These recent developments indicate that community

agencies will have to adapt generic need assessment methodologies in identifying and studying the needs of specialized populations, as well as in assessing the needs of the community at large.

## NOTES

1.  Community mental health centers amendments of 1975, Title III, Public Law 94–63.

2.  Windle, C., & Ochberg, F. Enhancing program evaluation in the community mental health centers program. *Evaluation*, 1975, *2*, 30–36.

3.  The national health planning and resources development act of 1974. Public Law 93–641; 93rd Congress S.2994, January 4, 1975.

4.  Tripodi, T., Fellin, P., & Epstein, I. *Social program evaluation: Guidelines for H.E.W. administrators.* Itasca, Ill.: Peacock Publishers, 1971.

5.  Sundel, M. *Introducing an evaluation program in an evolving regional human services delivery system.* Paper presented at the Southeastern Psychological Association, New Orleans, April 1973.

6.  Warheit, G., Bell, R., & Schwab, J. *Planning for change: Needs assessment approaches.* Rockville, Md.: National Institute of Mental Health, 1974.

7.  Goldsmith, H. F., & Unger, E. L. *Social areas: Identification procedures using 1970 census data.* (Laboratory Paper No. 37). Mental Health Studies Center, NIMH, May, 1972.

8.  Morrison, B. J., & Sundel, M. Development of a community assessment strategy for program evaluation in a comprehensive human service delivery system. In J. Zusman & C. Wurster (Eds.), *Program evaluation: Alcohol, drug abuse, and mental health services.* Lexington, Mass.: D.C. Heath, 1975.

9.  Redick, R. W., Goldsmith, H. F., & Unger, E. L. *1970 census data used to indicate areas with different potential for mental health and related problems* (Mental Health Statistics Series C, No. 3). NIMH, 1971.

10.  Rosen, B. M. *A model for estimating mental health needs using 1970 census socio-economic data* (DHEW Publication No. (ADM) 74–63), 1974.

11.  Rosen, B. M., Lawrence, L., Goldsmith, H., & Windle, C. *Mental health demographic profile system description* (DHEW Publication No. (ADM) 76–263), 1976.

12.  Sundel, M. The development and implementation of program and facility standards in a comprehensive community mental health program: A case in point. In R. H. Heighton (Ed.), *State mental health standards: How to do it.* Atlanta, Georgia: Southern Regional Education Board, 1976.

13.  Sundel, M., & Schanie, C. Community mental health and mass media preventive education: The Alternatives project. *Social Service Review*, 1978, *52*, 297–306.

14.  Padilla, A. M., Ruiz, R. A., & Alvarez, R. Community mental health services for the Spanish surnamed population. *American Psychologist*, 1975, *30*, 892–905.

15.  Gurin, G., Veroff, J., & Feld, S. *American view their mental health* (Joint Commission on Mental Illness and Health, Monograph Series No. 4). New York: Basic Books, 1960.

16.  Hughes, C. C., Tremblay, M., Rapoport, R. H., & Leighton, A. H. *People of cove and woodlot* (Vol. II. The Stirling County study). New York: Basic Books, 1960.

17.  Langner, T. S., & Michael, S. T. *Life stress and mental health: The Midtown Manhattan study* (Vol II). Glencoe, Ill.: Free Press, 1963.

18.  Leighton, D. C. The distribution of psychiatric symptoms in a small town. *American Journal of Psychiatry*, 1956, *112*, 716–723.

19.  Leighton, A. H. *My name is legion* (Vol. I. The Stirling County study). New York: Basic Books, 1959.

20.  Leighton, D., Harding, J., Macklin, D., Macmillan, A., & Leighton, A. *The character of danger* (Vol. III. The Stirling County study). New York: Basic Books, 1963.

21.  Schwab, J. J., & Warheit, G. J. Evaluating southern mental health needs and services. *Florida Medical Journal*, 1972, *59*, 17–20.

22.  Srole, L., Lagner, T., Michael, S., Opler, J., & Rennie, T. *Mental health in the metropolis* (Vol I. The Midtown Manhattan study). New York: McGraw-Hill, 1962.

23.  Bell, R. A., Keeley, K., Clemens, R., Warheit, G., & Holzer, C. Alcoholism, life events, and psychiatric impairment. *New York Academy of Science*, 1976, *237*, 467–480.

24. Bylaws of Kentucky Region Eight Mental Health-Mental Retardation Board, Inc. Louisville, Kentucky, 1966. Article 2, Section I.

25. Sundel, M. *Introducing and developing a goal-oriented record keeping system in a regional human services program.* Paper presented at a workshop on program evaluation for administrators, Los Angeles, California, July 1973.

26. *Survey of mental health needs in Kentucky.* Louisville, Kentucky: Kentucky Association for Mental Health and Kentucky Psychiatric Association, 1972.

27. Jahoda, M. *Current concepts of positive mental health.* New York: Basic Books, 1960.

28. Sells, S. B. (Ed.). *The definition and measurement of mental health* (Public Health Service Pub. No. 1873). Washington, D.C.: U.S. Department H.E.W., 1968.

29. Sundel, M., & Sundel, S. *Behavior modification in the human services: A systematic introduction to concepts and applications.* New York: John Wiley, 1975.

30. Kish, L. *Survey sampling.* New York: John Wiley, 1965.

31. Joint Commission on Accreditation of Hospitals (JCAH). *Principles for the accreditation of community mental health centers* (working draft). Division of Community Mental Health of the Accreditation Council for Psychiatric Facilities, December 15, 1975.

32. Turner, J. C., & TenHoor, W. J. The NIMH Community Support Program: Pilot approach to a needed social reform. *Schizophrenia Bulletin,* 1978, *4,* 319–348.

33. The President's Commission on Mental Health. *Report to the President from the President's Commission on Mental Health* (Vol. I). Washington, D.C.: Superintendent of Documents, U.S. Government Printing Office, 1978.

*Chapter 15*

# PROCEDURES FOR MAXIMIZING USAGE OF NEED ASSESSMENT DATA

## *Stanley A. Murrell*

The basic premise here is that any need assessment project should be judged against two equally important criteria. A successful need assessment project must both: (1) provide information collected via unbiased methods and (2) provide information that is subsequently used in program operations. Please note: this basic premise places responsibility for the *usage* of need assessments directly on the need assessor.

This chapter will focus on the usage criterion since in my view the conversion process has been comparatively neglected. However, this does not reflect a position that *usage* is more important than unbiased data, only that it is equally important. The procedures for usage follow.

### STEP 1: HAVE PATIENCE AND TAKE A LONG-TERM TIME PERSPECTIVE

Data people tend to be in a hurry to collect the data. They "get off" on data and can hardly wait to see them. They have a tendency to want to get the data and then go on to another project. They have a tendency to "report and run." Program people, on the other hand, tend to have a longer view, certainly beyond any one need assessment project. To work better together, assessors need to have a mental set that the project extends considerably beyond the data collection phase.

The need assessor should be prepared to spend a great deal of time simply getting to know the manager and the sponsor organization *before* the need assessment project is designed. This time may well "feel" unproductive, but it is necessary in order to obtain an estimate of the benefits-to-risk ratio of the need assessment to the organization and thereby gearing the project to maximum usage.

The need assessor should also be prepared to spend a great deal of time with the sponsor *after* the data has been collected: in data analysis, data interpretation, application activities, and new project development.

The Denver Research Institute of the University of Denver has reported its analysis of six need assessment projects[1] with a particular focus on utilization. For usage, it recommends arrangements that provide continued involvement beyond data collection.

It is appropriate for the sponsor to expect and demand that postcollection procedures be planned and specified in advance.

## STEP 2: DO AN ASSESSMENT OF THE SPONSOR

In the present context, we will assume the sponsor has already decided to have some form of need assessment. The question is whether he will use the data after collection.

A guiding principle is as follows: the degree to which need assessment data is converted into program operations is some function of the sponsor's perception of the ratio of assessment benefits to its risks. At the very outset of a need assessment project, in the initial discussions of the kind of need information to be collected, it can be expected that the sponsor will, at least intuitively, apply the benefit-to-risk ratio.

It seems to follow from this guiding principle that before need assessors do anything else, a "diagnosis" of the organization is required.

Many of us have learned in our direct service work that a referral problem cannot simply be accepted at face value. For example, in the mental health area the original referral problem may be a child's behavior in school, yet after closer examination and more information the child's behavior turns out to be less serious than other problems in the family, for example, marital problems between the parents. In the same way, a stated desire by a sponsor organization to "do a need assessment" cannot be taken simply at face value. If the usage criterion is taken seriously, the ostensible desire must be diagnosed by first assessing the sponsor. What does the sponsor really want, and what would make him or her really apprehensive? After all, information can be dangerous: it can bankrupt a company, drive a person to suicide, force a president to resign, etc. Information can force change. In order to optimize the chances of the information being converted into program operations, the assessor needs to know the sponsor's real perceptions.

After doing an assessment and determining benefits and risks, we would need to estimate the impact of the need assessment project on the sponsor. As an example of this, I will suggest possible risks to sponsors of different need assessment techniques. The point here is to emphasize that sponsor characteristics will interact with need assessment *procedures* at all phases and that the consequences will affect the conversion process.

## Nominal Group Technique

Delbecq and Van de Ven[3] have devised a five-stage process, leading from problem identification by citizens through to program operation, in one of the few methods that explicitly deals with the conversion of data into program operations. The first stage they have named the nominal group technique. A cross-section of community citizens is brought together and broken down into small groups. Then, through a highly structured, task-directed procedure, the citizens provide their ideas as to problems and priorities, both individually and in groups. The research shows that this technique maximizes both generation of ideas and individual satisfaction, and prevents unrepresentative predominance by a few individuals (see Chapter 12).

From a sponsor's point of view this could be a high-risk

method. The sponsor cannot control the inputs from the citizens. Specific risk "hot spots" cannot be avoided in advance. All sorts of "surprise" data and priorities may arise, and they become public immediately. A sponsor using such a method must have a strong ideological commitment to following citizen priorities rather than organizational or professional priorities. Sponsors with very high risk-tolerance would enjoy this method, those with low risk-tolerance would be scared by it.

## Social Indicators Technique

This term includes a whole family of approaches variously named: demographic analysis, ecological analysis, social area analysis, etc. This technique uses population-level data. The most typically used data in this technique is that of the Census Bureau, for example, the demographic profiles that are available for community mental health agency catchment areas (MHDP), as described by Redick, Goldsmith, and Unger[4] and Goldsmith and Unger.[5] These data are indirect indices of needs or problems. Correlates of these data with health and mental health indices have been found[6] (see Chapter 8).

For the sponsor, there is some potential risk in using social indicators. There is no control over the data itself, leaving uncertainty. With census data, the measures are so standard and have become familiar to so many people that it would be difficult to steer around specific risk "hot spots" to safer areas. On the other hand, since these measures are well known, the sponsor can have a better idea in advance of the kinds of information it will be getting; surprises are less likely than in the nominal group approach.

For any technique, degree of perceived risk depends a great deal upon the purpose for which the information will be used. If social indicators were to be used as base line data against which to evaluate program impact, this could pose a considerable risk to a program since such measures are presumably the result of so many and such pervasive social forces, and they are such gross measures, that they might not be sensitive to real program impact. The program's existence could be threatened, and in this case unfairly.

Less risky, but still of concern, would be the use of the social indicators as a standard against which to compare the user population in order to identify underserved subpopulations, that is, if 11 percent of the population is 65 or older but only 2 percent of the agency's clients are 65 or older, then this age group may be underserved by this agency. Such comparisons might strongly call for change: for new kinds of services, or new locations for services.

Still less risk would be involved in using social indicators to identify high need geographical areas within a community. Based on previous work, the assessor can have a good idea of the outcome of such a project. There would be few surprises.

## Field Survey Technique

The nominal group approach is something like shooting a large gauge shotgun; you are not sure what you might hit. The social indicators technique is perhaps a smaller gauge shotgun whose risk depends on the target. By comparison, the field survey is a rifle. The particular need area can be precisely specified by the items asked. With the field survey, the assessor can aim accurately at usable questions without danger of hitting risky topics.

Actually, it is more precise to say that the field survey is more adjustable to risk-tolerance. By item selection, the survey can be aimed very specifically, or through open-ended questions it could be very exploratory and then turn up unanticipated information. However, the critical consideration, for the sponsor's risk-tolerance, is that this adjustment can be planned.

A different type of risk is posed by the field survey, and, ironically, it is posed by the survey's strongest methodologic advantage. As an applied research method, the survey can give the most representative information (assuming sampling is properly executed) for the target population. Any one respondent's answers are equal to those of any other. The voice of any sub-group is proportional to its number in the general population. The data are unweighted. The sponsor, however, may not be able to afford to rely exclusively on the representative, but unweighted, data of surveys. County commissioners, for example, may see the need priorities of the county very differently from those reflected in a survey; but their opinions might have to be given more weight if their opinions would influence the agency's funding.

A sponsor might need to avoid being caught between these two sources of data. Similarly, the health and human service problems of a community do not have an equivalent impact on all citizens of that community. Physicians, ministers, judges, and school principals, for example, feel the impact of mental health problems much more directly than the average survey respondent. "Feelings of dissatisfaction" might be the most frequently reported mental health symptom by respondents in a survey; however "drug abuse," affecting a much smaller percentage of the population, actually has a much more intense, much stronger impact on the community.

The survey tells the story in terms of unweighted frequencies. The sponsor must also have influence-weighted information if it is that information that determines its maintenance inputs. Still, in general, the survey appears to pose less risk than either the nominal group or social indicators technique.

## Key Informants

In contrast to the unweighted data of the survey, this approach provides just such information. Interviews with selected key people (such as county commissioners, ministers, and principals) give useful information on impact of problems. This is typically rather safe data for a sponsor organization since a social service or health agency will usually be in the same ideological network with such key informants, and surprises are unlikely. Also, such key informants are not likely to go out of their way to be critical of the sponsor organization.

## Rates-Under-Treatment Technique

The rates-under-treatment approach, also referred to as the client utilization approach, uses information about current usage of services to estimate need. In the most basic descriptive sense, these data report numbers and characteristics of people seen for services. For many service agencies this type of information is routinely required in some form (see Chapter 9).

When used alone, this approach would provide little threat

to most sponsors. There is little pressure exerted for change because the data only report what has been done. Also, most service agencies can use these data to show increasing usage of and need for their services, which can then be used as evidence for the need for increased levels of maintenance inputs. However, if usage of services were sharply on the decline, these data could pose problems for an agency. From the sponsor's perspective, the data are well controlled; there is little uncertainty or potential for surprises. Used alone this technique is unlikely to run into sensitive areas. In short, this technique appears in general to pose the least risk of the four methods discussed to this point.

## Dynamic Modeling Technique

The above five techniques are established and well known. However, as this whole "data-for-decisions" movement continues to grow, we can expect refinements and additional, more ambitious techniques to be used. One of these may be the dynamic modeling technique, which has been tested by Newbrough and Christenfeld[7] as part of their feasibility study for monitoring the depressed mood of a community. The researchers used dynamic modeling to see whether they could predict the mood level of a community using monthly indices for a span of 60 months. These indices included such community level measures as divorce rates, unemployment rates, death rates, etc., over the 60 months.

Dynamic modeling derives from work done by Jay Forrester[8] who has used computer simulation to study the dynamics of different very large complex systems, including such relationships as those between housing and employment under urban renewal. The basic idea of this technique is to simulate what has happened in the past via computer to build a model for use in predicting what will happen in the future.

Newbrough's evaluation was that the technique showed great promise but pointed to the need for added and better measures related to resources and positive outcomes in addition to those which relate to problems. That is, we have measures established as being related to such events as hospital admissions, but do not have measures established as being related to hospital discharges.[6] What happens in the community to influence improvement? Are such measures as availability of social networks or follow-up service programs related to hospital discharge?

Dynamic modeling basically takes the social indicator approach and "rolls" it over time. The social indicator, as now most frequently used, is a static procedure. The dynamic modeling technique, therefore, first possesses the modest risk-potential of the social indicator approach and adds the risks inherent in not knowing what relationships will be found over time. Initially, then, until such models become well established and we know more about what to expect, this must be considered a high-risk technique suitable only for sponsors with a high risk-tolerance.

## STEP 3: COLLABORATION WITH THE SPONSOR: SPECIFY THE CHOICE-POINTS

It should be remembered that up to this point the design for the need assessment has not yet even been started. The design begins at this point: the assessor should confer with sponsors about their program decisions.

In these conferences, assessors should accomplish certain things: (1) they should lay out their information about the sponsor gained from the organizational assessment; (2) the sponsor leaders should be asked to respond to this assessment to clarify, to criticize, to agree, or to disagree; (3) hopefully a consensus perception of the sponsor organization should emerge (if there is not complete accord, at least each knows what the other knows, there is a common base of information); (4) an agreement as to the real benefits and risks should be reached, and sponsors should be asked to indicate the relative importance of those benefits and risks; (5) after these prior steps, a written delineation of the decisions-to-be-made and choice-points should be developed through collaboration. These written choice-points should specify the different program alternatives for which information is needed.

Generally, up to a point, the more specific the choice-points, the more relevant will be the need assessment information. The Denver Institute[1] suggests the advantages for usage of having a specific program focus. However, it is even more important, as is also noted by the Denver Institute, for the overall plan to be user-based. That is, the information collected must be congruent with the requirements of the sponsor if it is to be used. Thus, for data concerns, the more specific the better, but the choice-points must be defined by sponsor terms first, and the assessor should not pressure for more specificity than the sponsor is willing or able to give. Too much pressure for specificity, for reducing sponsor choice-points to measurable units, may merely lead to concerns that are trivial or artificial for the sponsor. This would give the data less visible relevance, which would then lead perhaps to low utilization.

It is recommended that at this stage the focus be exclusively on the program alternatives and decisions. Method and measurement decisions should not be introduced before the choice-points are clarified. Purpose should dictate method, method should not dictate purpose. However, in the next step the realities of method must be directly confronted.

## Step 4: The Assessor Selects the Method

In this step, usage considerations must take a back seat to methodologic and measurement considerations.

First, the assessor must judge the choice-points and purposes as defined in the prior step to be legitimate and appropriate and feasible for a need assessment. If the purposes are not acceptable to the assessor, the assessor should not proceed with the need assessment.

Next, if the purposes are acceptable, the assessor should then specify the appropriate techniques and data to be collected. This decision is not negotiable. It is the exclusive responsibility of the assessor to insure unbiased information.

Next, the assessor should describe the selected techniques and their potential yields to the sponsor. The risks and benefits to the sponsor, insofar as the assessor knows them, should be specified and clearly communicated to the sponsor in advance.

Then, having this information, the sponsor has the option of deciding against doing the need assessment. There is no major loss if the sponsor does decide to call it off. A need assessment the sponsor does not want will receive little use and is therefore not successful.

The assessor does not have the option of compromising data to accommodate sponsor apprehensions. Nor does the assessor have the option of compromising the data to better fit his or her *own* hidden agendas. Any assessor may be an advocate for or against certain programs or practices. Merely holding such opinions is not a problem as long as they are explicit and do not bias the data. My view is that need assessments should never be used as *covert* interventions by assessors.

### STEP 5: PLAN FOR MAXIMUM FLEXIBILITY IN THE FORM OF THE DATA

The Denver Institute reported that data accessibility was closely related to its usage. It is suggested here that as the need assessment project is being designed, the accessibility and the flexibility of the *form* of the data be carefully considered. For example, collecting and storing datum in its smallest possible unit allows for later reclassification, for example, coding data by census block rather than census tract would allow for a more fine-grained analysis of a geographical area. Using the same boundaries as other social indicator data improves the possibility of comparing areas. The more comprehensive the identification or coding, the more retrievable the data are for different analysis and the more flexible its use.

As much as possible, then, data flexibility should be built into the design. It is recognized that all possible uses cannot be fully anticipated; however, the more flexible and accessible the data, the more possible it will be to accommodate future usage.

### STEP 6: PLAN FOR POST-DATA PROCEDURES

It is suggested here that as the need assessment is being designed, the application procedures be planned in detail. To insure that the information necessary for usage is in fact collected, it is important to plan in advance for the application of data to program operations. Without this detailed advance planning, there is the danger of failing to collect that information most critical for application. Planning for this usage directs the assessor to the information that will be needed. Such planning should obviously be in collaboration with sponsor staff.

For example, one might prepare by actually writing up a report before the data are collected, using dummy data, anticipating different possible results, and then detailing the implications of those different results for program applications. Clearly, program people would be involved in this exercise. The discipline of putting words, ideas, and program activities down on paper in this manner may help to identify the kind of data necessary for program application.

Planning for application in advance also helps to establish the set for both assessor and sponsor that application procedures are an integral part to be included within the need assessment project. This may prevent tendencies by some assessors to "report and run."

It may also be useful at this stage to work out the ground rules for resolving differences regarding data analysis and data interpretation. For example, data sometimes may be interpreted with opposing implications if the program people see it one way and the data people see it another. What should be the ground rules for resolving and reporting these differences?

During this step, anticipating usage implications, the design for the need assessment project is completed. Data are then collected. Now to the next step after data collection.

### STEP 7: INVOLVE SPONSOR IN DATA ANALYSIS AND DATA INTERPRETATION

This is a tricky step. It is a step where the data criterion and the usage criterion are about equally balanced. Many of us in this need assessment field are in it because data "turn us on." The data seduce us. There is a special excitement to seeing the data "hot" out of the computer. To promote usage, it is desirable to expose the users to this data excitement early, to have them "get their hands in."

For example, it is beneficial to have program people suggest items to "cross-tab" or to suggest population breakdowns for certain items. Program people will "see" useful questions to ask of data because of their familiarity with the populations, programs, and geographical areas, and this involvement helps them to become familiar and confident with the assessment data.

The Denver Institute reports that this involvement by users in data analysis and interpretation contributed strongly to utilization in several of the projects they studied. However, they also note that program people may have such strong biases that they are unable to interpret the data appropriately. This seems to suggest that program people, compared to data people, either have stronger biases or are more likely to introduce their biases into the data interpretation. Whether this is indeed accurate, or whether it may reflect a bias of "us data people," is unclear at this time. However, there clearly could be a problem that would weaken either one or the other of the two criteria for need assessment success. This is why it is important to establish ground rules before data collection in advance.

During this stage, the data are applied, new programs are planned, old programs are redesigned, resources are redistributed, etc., utilization occurs. But need assessment should not end.

## STEP 8: BEGIN PLANNING FOR NEXT NEED ASSESSMENT

This is the eighth step but should not be the end of the need assessment. The data itself and the process of applying data will raise new questions and point to needs for added information. The period of data analysis, data interpretation, and data utilization is a fertile period for planning further data collection. Need assessment should not come to an end; it should be a continuous, ongoing process. Utilization then helps guide the next data collection project.

As is true with methodologic procedures, in actual practice the complete accomplishment of each of these usage procedures will not be possible. However, the continued neglect of usage considerations will not only lead to more unsuccessful need assessment projects but will also lead to a rejection of the general need assessment approach to program improvement (e.g., Kimmel[9]). After all, the purpose is better programs.

## FUTURE DIRECTIONS FOR NEED ASSESSMENT

I will close this chapter with some guesses about the future. I think the present gaps that separate program people from data people will continue to be narrowed. I believe data people will become less arrogant and self-righteous; program people will become less defensive and fixed in their ways. The training of both will improve to aid each in understanding the language of the other. Close harmony is probably not possible, perhaps not even desirable; but I think working relationships will continue to improve.

Areas outside health and human resources will increasingly contribute to an expanding repertoire of need assessment methods. For example, the field of environmental design has produced some fascinating work on *trade-off game* methods, wherein the respondent is asked to make choices with differential "costs" (see Robinson et al.[10]). Such an approach shows promise for citizen participation in government resource allocation.

I believe need assessment will grow larger than the health and human service fields. Already, the basic idea and some of the methods are being used by government at different levels (e.g., Urban Studies Center[11]). Across the country, there is now an increasing interest in whether field surveys of citizen priorities can be used by local government for budget-making, as shown in the work of Hatry and Blair,[12] Jackson and Shade,[13] and Murrell and Shulte.[14]

As need assessment grows up, it will be given greater responsibilities. If it continues to play an increasing role in money allocations, it will become even more of a power tool. If its power potentials increase, appropriate application will come under even greater pressure to withstand attempts to influence the data. Need assessment activities will increasingly need to be protected from misuse and misrepresentation at the same time that they will increasingly need to be converted to program operations.

## NOTES

1.  Denver Research Institute. *Analysis and synthesis of needs assessment research in the field of human services.* Denver, Colorado: Denver Research Institute Publication, 1974.

2.  Berrien, F. K. *General and social systems.* New Brunswick, N. J.: Rutgers University Press, 1968.

3.  Delbecq, A. L., & Van de Ven, A. A group process model for problem identification and program planning. *Journal of Applied Behavioral Science,* 1971, *7,* 466–492.

4.  Redick, R. W., Goldsmith, H., & Unger, E. L. *1970 census data used to indicate areas with different potentials for mental health and related problems.* (National Institute of Mental Health Statistics Methodology Reports, Series C., No. 3). Washington, D.C.: U.S. Govt. Printing Office, 1971.

5.  Goldsmith, H., & Unger, E. L. *Social areas: Identification procedures using 1970 census data.* (Laboratory Paper No. 37). Adelphi, Md.: Mental Health Study Center, National Institute of Mental Health, 1972.

6.  Bloom, B. An ecological analysis of psychiatric hospitalizations. *Multivariate Behavioral Research,* 1968, *3,* 423–464.

7.  Newbrough, J. R., & Christenfeld, R. M. *Community mental health epidemiology: Nashville.* Final report of NIMH Grant Project, No. MH-206681, 1975.

8.  Forrester, J. W. *Urban dynamics.* Cambridge, Mass.: The M.I.T. Press, 1969.

9.  Kimmel, W. *Needs assessment: A critical perspective.* (Office of Program Systems, Office of the Assistant Secretary for Planning and Evaluation, Department of Health, Education and Welfare), 1977.

10.  Robinson, I. M., Baer, W. C., Banerjee, T. K., & Flachsbart, P. G. Trade-off games. In W. Michelson (Ed.), *Behavioral research methods in environmental design.* Stroudsburg, Pa.: Dowden, Hutchinson & Ross, 1975.

11.  Urban Studies Center. *Community priorities and evaluations.* (Vols. 1–15). Louisville: Urban Studies Center, University of Louisville, 1974–79.

12.   Hatry, H. & Blair, L. Citizen surveys for local governments: A cop out, manipulative tool, or policy guidance and analysis aid? In T. N. Clark (Ed.), *Citizen preferences and urban public policy*. Beverly Hills, Calif.: Sage, 1976.

13.   Jackson, J. S. III & Shade, W. Citizen participation, democratic representation, and survey research. *Urban Affairs Quarterly*, 1973, *9*, 57–89.

14.   Murrell, S. & Schulte, P. A procedure for systematic citizen input to community decision-making. *American Journal of Community Psychology*, 1980, *8*, 19–30.

*Chapter 16*

# TRANSLATING NEED ASSESSMENT AND RESOURCE IDENTIFICATION DATA INTO HUMAN SERVICE GOALS

## Harold W. Demone

Contemporary American human services planning is characterized by two major themes: (1) citizen participation and (2) increasing use of technology. For example, the computer must be recognized as a highly significant technological advance which permits the development of sophisticated information systems from which health and welfare indicators can be refined. A number of related projects are now occurring at local and national levels, and the possibility of technologically determined rationality looms on the horizon. In principle, we can for the first time control many of the significant variables and simulate complex social experiments. Our faith can be reinforced by the rationality of machine as against the infinite potential perfidy of man. The citizen participation movement, however, does provide a distinct compensatory mechanism.

The application of technologically derived data is also increasingly sophisticated. Planners are using tools such as performance and program budgets for comparative analysis; management information systems are increasingly being implemented; accrual accounting will soon be standard; and other controlled data collection techniques and analytic frameworks are providing new guidelines to policy making and problem solving.[1]

Developmentally, planning seems to have achieved a plateau. Although we have substantially capitalized on the current technology of accounting, biostatistics, and economics, additional breakthroughs are necessary. These gains probably should be generated increasingly from the social sciences, for example, sociology, anthropology, psychology, and political science.

Within this state of affairs, the human services planner focuses on four areas: policy making, problem solving, and interorganizational and intraorganizational relations. Within each area, five subgoals can be identified to make services: (1) more available, (2) more accessible, (3) more continuous, (4) cost effective, and (5) of improved quality. The superordinate objective is to prevent the occurrence of the problem. The most meaningful gains are likely to be in the policy area, an area dominated at the public level by the legal profession, although economics has made some gains in the last decade. With its focus on resource optimization, economics has credibility and nonideological potential. It can analyze the cost-benefits of state-imposed "workfare" programs and determine that costs exceed benefits. Simultaneously, the Administration and Congress and their state-level peers can ignore the findings and impose nonfunctional statutory requirements. Clearly, our elected officials are not convinced that a scientific discipline has any unique competence to contribute to goal formulation, although much of the controversy within economics has to do with just that question. Kecskemeti[2] would agree with the politicians. He suggests that goals are not neutral, not impartial, and not truly measurable; thus they are not scientific. It is the inevitable existential nature and consequent compromises of policy that limit the contributions of both scientists and planners.

One increasingly popular technology is the needs-resource study. For example, Title XX of the Social Security Act specifically requires an annual plan and highlights the importance of needs studies. The Community Mental Health and Health Planning Acts also speak encouragingly of needs-resource studies.

In specifying such requirements, it is unclear whether the Congress and the bureaucracy are merely asking us to demonstrate that our efforts are based on more than tradition and intuition, or are encouraging the application of more rigorous data collection and analytic methods and more sophisticated theories.

The significant issue is that today's critical problems are not amenable to straightforward solutions. Reducing the rates of alcoholism, substance abuse, or mental illness is exponentially more difficult than improving the quality of water in a rural area. The rate of diminishing return is a hard taskmaster.

Let me now describe some of my own experiences and extrapolate from them. In reflecting back over more than 20 years, I am surprised to find that despite my general cynicism about the effective use of data in policy making and problem solving, I have been considerably involved in such efforts with some modestly successful results. Need assessment studies in alcoholism, mental retardation, and fluoridation are some of the examples that come to mind. I will describe these experiences to illustrate how the policy planning practitioner attempts to use data and some of the results of these efforts.

## CASE EXAMPLES

### Needs-Resource Data Utilization in Alcoholism

My first intensive experience with need studies was in the 1950s when I headed up alcoholism programs in two different states. Organized treatment resources were scanty; Alcoholics Anonymous provided the bulk of the services. Estimates of the size of the population at need, compared to the available resources, were political necessities. How could we compete effectively with those touting the incidence of tuberculosis, crime, mental illness, heart disease, or cancer without our own scorecard? Fortunately, alcoholism had a brilliant biostatistician, E. M. Jellinek, who developed a formula based upon reported deaths from cirrhosis of the liver. The formula is still in widespread use although Jellinek urged, almost two decades ago, that its continued use be stopped. Clearly, political necessities still abound.

In fact, when the alcoholics then in custody of public organizations were totaled, they substantially exceeded all those in treatment in Alcoholics Anonymous and alcoholism clinics combined. Demand substantially exceeded capacity. Thus, even the conservative measure of an actual current body count of individuals with a primary or secondary diagnosis of alcoholism or an arrest for chronic public drunkenness provided an overwhelming number of potential clients. Thus, I began to use two sets of needs data—the number as determined by the Jellinek formula and the number in formal contact with various agencies. As for utilization of the data by my bosses in the Executive Branch or the Legislature, the gap, by either needs identification method, was so great that we threatened rather than encouraged them.

At a budget writing session held by the Governor with his small group of senior trusted colleagues, my alcoholism program request was in review. My Jellinek-calculated number of alcoholics was noted. One of those present concluded reasonably that "Demone was crazy." General agreement seemed to occur until one of those present mused out loud about the three or four alcoholics that he knew. This stimulated similar analysis. Each person present knew personally one or more alcoholics. That an extrapolation of their data method would have given a total number of alcoholics two or three times the total state population was fortunately not concluded! The net result was that I regained some lost credibility and a recommendation for a small increase in our annual operating budget.

Data can be overwhelming and challenge some of our most cherished beliefs. Continuing with alcoholism for the moment, paralleling the Joint Commission on Mental Illness, a national Cooperative Commission on Alcoholism, of which I was the commissioner, operated from 1960 to 1966. On one occasion, we updated the Jellinek formula estimate for California, agreed on a nominal number of annualized outpatient visits per client, giving a total number of clinical hours necessary for all of California's alcoholics. As you might guess, all the psychiatrists, clinical psychologists, and psychiatric social workers in the United States would not have been sufficient to treat the alcoholics in California. Even more discouraging is that carefully designed and administered household surveys conducted locally, regionally, and nationally over the last decade or so tend to produce a number of problem drinkers often in excess of that determined by the Jellinek formula. So, our problem is apparently not a bias toward overestimation. What many reasonable observers have concluded is that the solution to the problem of alcoholism is not to be found in the singular expansion of specialized alcoholism treatment facilities. Instead, strengthening of the capacity and willingness of the generic caregiving system and emphasis on primary and secondary prevention are the current policy choices. Thus, for alcoholism, at least, needs-resources analyses have influenced public policy to some degree.

## Need Assessment in Mental Retardation

As a consequence of the normal curve, about 3 percent of the population will have an IQ score of below 70. Similarly, the schools generally find the same proportion needing special services and/or education. It would be easy, therefore, for mental retardation planners to assume that lifetime services for the retarded should be developed for 3 percent of the population, and many recommend programs to that effect. But a valid diagnosis of mental retardation requires measures of general adaptation in addition to intellectual impairment. Furthermore, both must be present and have developed prior to mental maturity (age 17). When you realize that the hardest measure is the often criticized IQ test, it should be clear that the classical needs-measurement procedure in retardation has some weaknesses. Before I describe some of our experiences with this measure, I will give you my conclusion, which is generally shared by most sophisticated observers of retardation.[3] Prevalence studies are unnecessary and wasteful because we already know the distribution of intelligence in the general population. Furthermore, there is minimal correlation between IQ scores and adult social adjustment.

Why do I feel we no longer need prevalance studies and what do we do instead? First of all, most retardates—at least 75 percent—are diagnosed as such because of psychosocial disadvantages; this differentiation is most prominent during school ages when a captive audience is available for measurement. Our mid-1960s follow-up study of all educable males who terminated their special class education in about 200 separate school systems in Massachusetts over a two-year period shows that 85 percent had been working steadily during the subsequent five-year period.[4]

Their general occupational and social adjustment was about the same as their siblings and peers of comparable age. Their major problem may well have been the school labeling process that they and their families fortunately tended to reject following school termination. The identifiable group with significant adjustment problems was the small percentage from upper and middle class families where expectation levels were unachievable. Prior to and after the school's labeling, 85 percent of these male "educable retardates" were using the normal service system and no lifetime special resources were necessary. The solution to sociocultural retardation is not in the hands of the retardation specialists since its origin lies in a mix of economic and social deprivation and linguistic handicaps. An increase in the minimum economic floor by a guaranteed annual income or some similar means would probably be the best avenue of attack.

This pattern of postschool adjustment means that organizationally we are talking about 20 to 25 percent of 3 percent (mostly those whom the schools call "trainable"), or less than 1 percent of the total population, who might need some special services. This is a more managable number and allows for the establishment of realistic goals.

From 1964 to 1966, I directed the Massachusetts Mental Retardation Planning Project.[5] Our responsibility was to develop a comprehensive 10-year plan for Massachusetts. Using the 3 percent calculation, there would have been 165,000 retardates living in Massachusetts (Table 16–1). A total of 34,514, or 20 percent of the possible 165,000, were identified by a statewide inventory in the last quarter of 1965. Of these, 12,255 were institutionalized in state schools, state hospitals for the mentally ill and epileptic, correctional institutions, and private residential homes. Of the remaining 22,289, over half were retarded persons in special classes. The others were on waiting lists for specialized retardation programs and in generic service or recreation programs (e.g., Boys' Clubs, Scouting). Thus, although we located about 34,500 of the estimated 165,000, slightly over one-third of those identified or 11,500, were found in the school system. Assuming again that the focus should be on the more

supporting direct services. The proposal, developed by staff, was discussed, amended, and refined by representatives of the major health, education, and welfare agencies of the state, each carefully scrutinizing it to guard against major abridgments of their autonomy.

Included on project task forces were members of the legislature, the state association for retarded children, and the state taxpayers association. The willingness of the bureaucrats to accept the proposal stemmed from recognition (reinforced by Project staff) that the Office of Retardation was an acceptable alternative to either transferring the retardation programs and facilities from one major state department to another, or developing an entirely new direct service agency.

The new office appeared to satisfy or at least pacify consumer group demands. For the first time, retardation was legitimized and programmed at the highest level of state government. The federal government adjudged the proposal to be innovative and provided matching support for the next five years. The Governor, in acknowledgement of the need and administrative complexity and with an eye to federal support, created the new office with minimum time lag. The legislature agreed, after some initial foot-dragging. Thus, a new office was created that, on hindsight, has been of reasonable value. This structural innovation represents one reasonable, yet limited, means toward meeting more general objectives. It was not the only alternative but appeared on balance to satisfy both substantive and strategic considerations at that time in Massachusetts. A client group would receive more planned and potentially more responsive services. The bureaucratic machinery serving this group was rationalized and opened to public scrutiny. It later served as the model for the first federal developmental disabilities legislation. A resource study had some effect on policy. (I would now recommend that a free standing direct service state agency be established for retardates).

*Citizen Participation in the Needs-Resource Decision-Making Process: Fluoridation*

An almost classic example of direct citizen determination of needs-resources can be seen by examining the flouridation controversy in this country from 1950 to date. It illustrates that discussions about citizens' participation in policy making and decision making neglect the process of referenda. Fluoridation is thus a scientific issue that has involved the direct participation of many voters in many communities across the country. It is not my intention to discuss the scientific background except to note that the cost of dental care is substantial and that fluoridation of water supply reduces dental decay, an affliction that almost all people suffer on many occasions during their lives. Further, according to Luther Terry,[7] former United States Surgeon General, it is one of the four major mass preventive health measures of all time. Thus, we have a relatively simple method that can substantially improve the health of most people at a very nominal cost. In addition, professional associations, public health authorities, presidents, and the World Health Organization have all called for the extension of fluoridation. Yet, when one examines the voting record of Americans over the period 1950 to 1966, the majority of communities (60 percent) voted *against* fluoridation of their water supply. As a fluoridation proponent during part of that period, I suffered my share of these defeats.

There are many explanations of this phenomenon. Crane and Rosenthal[8] classified the adopting and nonadopting communities by the structure of government. Fundamentally, those communities with strong leadership tended to adopt fluoridation by administrative action. Those with weak management and/or more democratic procedures were more likely to go through a referendum, with the results cited above.

There has been considerable research to determine why citizens would vote against something that is helpful, painless, and inexpensive. Two principal premises are offered. One is that people are generally alienated from their government, organized science, medicine, and the like. The alternative explanation is that since there had always been some physicians, dentists, and scientists who would oppose fluoridation and various impressive sounding organizations were established to embellish their opposition, the voters did not have a clear and informed choice.[9] Citizens witnessed confusion or disagreement between what appeared to them to be equally impressive scientific organizations and scientists. Generally, when people are uncertain, they vote against any such action on the correct assumption that they are merely postponing a decision and could later change their minds. Sapolsky concludes that they are not voting against fluoridation because of alienation, but because of confusion.

The other three significant public health measures mentioned by Luther Terry—pasteurization of milk, purification of water, and immunization against disease—were all adopted by administrative and legislative means. Summing up, Sapolsky noted: "Science does not advance by a show of hands and democracy cannot exist without citizen participation."[10] This conclusion, of course, leads us to such issues as the meaning of democracy, what is democratic, and whether citizen participation means choosing leaders to represent you or making judgments on each individual situation by referenda or other such means. Because we are in an era in which people increasingly want to participate and scientific innovations are increasingly complex, it is clear that we face existential questions. Perhaps the solution is the one advocated by Sapolsky, and that is to train our citizens to be able to deal with scientific arguments and scientific experts through an understanding of the limits and uses of science. Obviously, this recommendation is a long and not a short range solution. Sapolsky concludes pessimistically: "In the meantime, we may have to continue to forego the benefits of fluoridation and other similar innovations."[10]

The fluoridation findings are fascinating. The greater the citizen participation in the determination of resource utilization relative to need, the greater the likelihood that fluoridation will be rejected. Yet, surveys of the populations taken prior to or independently of the referendum campaigns showed an overwhelming pro-fluoridation stance. The ultimate irony was that the percentage supporting fluoridation was higher among those who did not understand its purpose than among those who correctly identified its function.[9]

## OBSTACLES TO UTILIZATION

### Planning Constraints

It is generally true that we tend simultaneously to overvalue our own profession and to be more aware of its limitation than outsiders. As such, it may be parochial for me as a planner to rationalize why our job is so difficult. Thus, I will quote J. T. O'Connor, a social scientist, to do it for me.[11] Speaking first of health planning as structured in 1966, he describes its operating environment as

> unfriendly and—probably more accurately—as hostile. Generally speaking, social planning has not been popular in any form in America. In a pluralistic and individualistic culture, this type of planning is seen as contrary to such revered traditions as individual freedom and the free enterprise system. Connoting regulation, coercion, forced interdependence, invasion of personal and institutional privacy, and disruption of the status quo, the concept of planning has always resurrected the typically American fear of excessive governmental intervention. The planning process assumes that those involved are ready to let some supra group decide what is best for them, and such a notion is relatively new to Americans.

But even worse in media-oriented America, the nature of effective planning for implementation often requires endless confidential negotiations with and between unwilling collaborators. Public discussions before, during, or after the planning process could be seriously inimical to the process and seriously impair the future credibility of a planning agency. As a rule of thumb, low visibility is the choice. The process requires great toleration for ambiguity, delay, and incremental achievements.

In addition to the environmental and process issues complicating the life of the planner, he is seldom trained to understand, interpret, evaluate, or apply research findings. The planner has been told that research, evaluation, continuing education, administration, and planning itself are all overhead items. By definition, overhead is to be reduced and controlled, ideally eliminated. And since a carefully designed research project will likely cost more than the experiment it is evaluating, it is unlikely that the planner will invest much of his limited resources on research.

## Research Constraints

David Truman suggests that the bearing of the social sciences on public policy has been a rocky one.[12] He reminds us of " . . . the gap between our aspirations or pretensions and our performance." He reminds us further as he looks ahead to the remainder of this century:

> Can policy be so taken as to provide moral choice among recognizable alternatives? These policies are not the domain of the social sciences, but it is reasonable to expect that these sciences should be able to offer substantial assistance in defining issues, shaping alternatives or interpreting consequences.

Nathan Caplan et al. classify the prevalent theories of utilization and nonutilization of social science findings in public policy formulation as: (1) knowledge, specific theories: (2) two-community theory; and (3) policy-maker-constraint theories.[13] Data from his study of 204 senior federal executive branch personnel, both civil service and political level appointees, led him to conclude that the Two-Community Theory accounts clearly for the bulk of observed variance. Thus, he concludes that underutilization is primarily a function "of a gap between social scientist and policy-makers due to difference in values, language, reward systems, and social and professional affiliations."[13] Caplan's Two-Community Theory suggests that political factors, time constraints, and the nature of desired information all combine to establish roles which limit opportunities to apply knowledge.

Although human service planners are appropriately impressed with the methodologic purity of much of social science research, they are hard pressed to identify findings applicable to their planning responsibilities. The entire American university research culture reinforces a certain trained incapacity by posing a fundamental conflict of interest for the researcher. Policy and problem-solving research is disvalued. And even if it were not, the federal research review procedure is counterproductive. The process takes years and thus is essentially a retrospective one for planners. Timely utilization is severely handicapped.

## WHEN NOT TO DO NEED-RESOURCE STUDIES

I will close this section on constraints with a list of don'ts, or when not to do need-resource studies. I will discuss the converse immediately following.

*Nature of the Data:*

Don't do the study when:

1. Your data, whatever the findings, would be irrelevant to critical policy or programmatic issues.
2. Your results will arrive too late for effective use.
3. The applications are politically unfeasible.
4. Your data lacks objectivity.
5. Methodologic weaknesses are evident.

*Capacity and Sophistication of the Researcher:*

Don't do the study when:

1. The likely findings conflict with your ideology, and you will find it difficult to remain objective.
2. You lack the capacity to disseminate and communicate the findings.
3. You are a political schmuck and lack politically sophisticated allies!

*Characteristics of Users:*

Don't do the study when:

1. The user is apathetic or strongly resistant to the use of such data. A corollary of this rule is to be cautious of organizations where support of influential vested interest groups has previously constrained their behavior.
2. The user population lacks the capacity to follow through.

3.  Users are more committed to values of intuition and experience than to science or empirical data.

Having noted these obstacles (and many more could be cited), you may still be willing to move ahead. The purposes may be of overwhelming concern or importance, and you have no ethical choice. If this is the case, you then have an equal responsibility to consider and include ways and means to overcome the problems, whatever they may be.

## Do Need-Resource Studies

*Nature of the Data:*

Do the study when:

1.  Efforts and resources can be concentrated on those need-resource questions for which it is feasible to secure meaningful answers.
2.  The findings would be relevant to decisions that are imminent regarding initiation, continuation, modification, or termination of a program.

## Conclusion

Having cautioned about the limits of data utilization in a real, complex, pluralistic, political, and competitive world, it is abundantly clear that more and improved data is necessary. At least, quantification may force definition and enhance open and honest debate about objectives. Comparisons are made possible.

Complementarily, as I note certain gross inadequacies in our ability to analyze alternatives effectively, we may only be a decade away from a new set of problems: that of data overload. The planner's future problem may not be the lack of data, but rather that of acquiring the skills to cope effectively with a surfeit of information. Expert opinion can be called upon to distinguish between the basic and surplus variables, but this approach often is insufficient, especially if citizen and consumer opinion is not given the same value as professional judgment.

Along with the many advantages posited for an age of technological planning, it is crucial that we also come to grips with its associated perils. The technology and language of planning are becoming increasingly complex, even at its present elementary stage. This escalating sophistication is going to make it increasingly complicated and difficult for even the well-educated nonplanner, professional, businessman, and community leader to participate effectively in decision making. Will this make them secure or insecure as objectively determined indices and solutions controvert politically reached solutions? If insecurity is fostered by the revision of priorities, the appropriateness of technological contributions will be increasingly questioned and perhaps even circumscribed.[1]

*Solutions*

As with all complex problems, there are no effective simple answers, but since recognition of the problem is necessary before solution, we can be said to be gaining. Part of the problem is attitudinal and part substantive.

Certainly, our graduate schools have the capacity to design training programs that educate researchers to comprehend policy and planning needs. An interdisciplinary stance is especially needed. Equally important, we need to train our researchers how to deal with resistance, how to truly "feel" the problem, and how to reward the use of data.

In addition, graduate programs in human services planning need a more scientific base. For the most part, they are still caught up in ideological struggles as to means and ends, processes and objectives.

Journals need to reconsider their policies in order to encourage more brief notes on findings and program implications rather than the continual seeking of methodological purity. Special attention should also be given to articles on policy considerations of research.

Need-resources studies and monitoring and descriptive research need to be tied more closely to the operating level. Researchers need to be linked to local agencies. The relation between user and researcher must be made inseparable.

Analysis must focus more often on the individual. We need a smaller scale social system focus. It will be more fruitful and productive.

Applied research needs more sanctions. It does not have to be nonconceptual; it can be generalized.

We need desperately to publicize negative results.

At the granting level, the federal government should specify research priorities more clearly. It might also consider experimental block grants that would encourage planning agencies to both engage in research and purchase task-oriented research skills.

At the local level, state and local governments, United Way organizations, and other bodies committed heavily to human service activities must be encouraged to invest more in the proactive rather than the almost exclusive thrust to reactive programs.

In conclusion, there is no single solution but a series of alternative available strategies, assuming we value rational decision making and believe the facts will enhance decision making.

## NOTES

1. Demone, H. W. and Schulberg, H. C. Planning for human services: The role of community councils. In H. W. Demone, Jr., and D. Harshbarger (Eds.), *A handbook of human service organizations.* New York: Behavioral Publications, 1973.

2. Kecskemeti, P. *Utilization of social research in shaping public policy.* Santa Monica: Rand Corporation, 1961.

3. Tarjan, G. *Mental retardation services.* Undated manuscript.

4. Mudd, M. Factors associated with the post school vocational adjustment of educable mental retarded boys in Massachusetts. Doctoral Dissertation, Brandeis University, 1968.

5. *Massachusetts plans for its retarded—a ten year plan.* Boston, Massachusetts: Medical Foundation, 1966.

6. Newman, E. and Demone, H. W., Jr. Policy paper; A new look at public planning for human services. *Journal of Health and Social Behavior,* 1969, *10,* 142–149.

7.  Terry, L. In *U.S. Public Health Service Emphasis.* Washington, D.C.: U.S. Government Printing Office, 1966.

8.  Crane, R. and Rosenthal, D. *The fluoridation decision, Report II, The community confronts an innovation.* Philadelphia: National Analysts, 1963.

9.  Sapolsky, H. M. Science, voters and the fluoridation controversy. *Science,* 1968, *162,* 427–433.

10. See Reference 9, p. 432.

11. O'Connor, J. T. Comprehensive health planning: Dreams and realities. *Health and Society,* 1974, *52,* 391–413.

12. Truman, D. B. The social sciences and public policy. *Science,* 1968, *162,* 162.

13. Caplan, N., Morrison, A., and Stambaugh, R. J. *The use of social science knowledge in policy decisions at the national level.* Ann Arbor, Michigan: Institute for Social Research, University of Michigan, 1975.

14. See Reference 13, p. 27.

Part V

# EPILOGUE ON NEED ASSESSMENT

## INTRODUCTION

It is difficult to arrive at a sense of closure in a field that is characterized by diverse constituencies, definitions, and methods. However, the first chapter in this section attempts such closure by reviewing the chapters of this volume and identifying both the state of the art and future directions for the field. Aponte clearly points out that there is much work to be done, particularly on conceptual and theoretical issues; methodology and strategy issues; and application, implementation, and utilization issues. A number of different disciplines and fields are capable of contributing to the clarification of these issues.

Aponte, Leone, and Bell conclude this section with an annotated bibliography. Included in this chapter are overviews and comprehensive readings; need assessment and planning; need assessment strategies, including the strategies described in this volume; utilization and application; examples of need assessments; and related readings. Familiarity with these readings should provide the reader with a critical understanding of need assessment in health and human services.

Chapter 17

# NEED ASSESSMENT

## The State of the Art and Future Directions*

## Joseph F. Aponte

The last five years have seen a growing interest and participation in the area of need assessment as evidenced by the increasing number of major publications and major conferences such as the First and Second National Conferences on Need Assessment in Health and Human Services held in Louisville, Kentucky. There are three primary reasons for this increased attention. First, recent legislation has mandated need assessment as a funding prerequisite for many programs, particularly those in health and human services. Second, there has been a recent emphasis on accountability and rational planning for service programs at federal, state, and local levels. Finally, the *zeitgeist* of our times requires sensitivity to recipient needs.

Over the past decade the amount of federal legislation on need assessment has grown. As Kimmel[1] points out, a need assessment is often a required part of the planning process or of the program plan, or a necessary precondition for grant support. Similarly, Zangwill,[2] in a detailed examination of Department of

*I would like to express my appreciation to Catherine Aponte and Elizabeth Lin for their editorial assistance on this chapter.

Health, Education, and Welfare programs referring to or requiring need assessment, found that (1) need assessment is required by law in almost half of the programs, (2) the regulations governing the other half also mandate need assessment, and (3) assessment results are typically a precondition for obtaining federal grants.

Of particular relevance is the passage of the National Health Planning and Resources Development Act of 1974 (PL 93–641) and the Health System Agency (HSA) established by this law. This agency, which coordinates regional, state, and national levels, has primary responsibility for planning, regulating, and developing local health resources. The extensive implications of this Act, which will potentially influence both need assessors and program people, include: (1) joint planning of mental and physical health services, (2) emphasis on service evaluation and regional planning, (3) increased consumer input in local level planning, and (4) greater availability of technical experts for planning services.[3,4]

The emphasis on rational service planning can be found everywhere. Constituents from all parts of the country, from all walks of life, and with varying levels of knowledge and expertise expect rational planning more than ever before. Service recipients, in particular, are demanding that health services meet their needs as effectively as possible. As then Senator Mondale succinctly put it:[5]

> We must, then, make choices—the best informed choices possible from the wealth of fragmented, scattered information we have in our possessions. We must design methods for filling the gaps in our information and methods to process such information systematically. We must develop a coherent set of problem definitions, goals, and solutions, and this is a task to be addressed at all levels of national life.

Such emphasis is indeed reflected at the national level. Peterson,[6] notes that three main themes have characterized the delivery of health care services: excellence, equity, and efficiency. The federal government is presently focusing on efficiency—with particular concern for establishing an equilibrium between rising health care costs and equal access to quality health care. This emphasis has encouraged the increased priority of program administrators and managers on rational decision making and planning. Finally, the zeitgeist of our times demands greater sensitivity to recipient needs. The service recipient, previously overlooked by planners and service providers, has begun to be conceptualized as an important element in the process. Schwab,[7] in this volume, notes that contributions to present interest and activities have been made by "humanitarian concerns, scientific pursuits, and compelling historical and social processes."[8] All of these forces have converged to make needs assessment a salient topic, particularly in the health and human services.

This chapter is divided into three major sections, reflecting both the organization of this volume and the literature in the field: (1) definitional and conceptual issues; (2) methodologic and strategy issues; and (3) application, implementation, and utilization issues. Each section can be examined independently, yet there are a number of issues and linkages across these broad areas. Implications for future directions in the field of health and human services need assessment will also be discussed.

## DEFINITIONAL AND CONCEPTUAL ISSUES

There are few uniformly accepted definitions of needs and need assessment.[1,9] A selected literature review indicates many different perspectives. For example, need assessments may be defined as systematic ways of identifying community needs; planning tools; data collecting and program planning methods; methods for establishing program priorities; methods for generating data in order to make administrative decisions; processes that allow for program decisions based on systematically collected data; and/or vehicles through which existing programs can be evaluated.[10–16] Consequently, difficulties have arisen in deriving common definitions. Specific assessment strategies that might be used to operationalize definitions have a variety of theoretical and conceptual bases, purposes, and objectives. Contributing to the confusion is the use of the term *need assessment* in at least two ways: as a generic term encompassing a variety of procedures or as a name for a single procedure. In this chapter, the term will be used generically, that is, to describe a variety of strategies that can be used to assess health and human needs.

Most of the focus has been on need assessment techniques, with little attention being paid to definitional and conceptual issues. Only recently have social scientists begun to direct their attention to these critical areas.[16–21] A review of the literature indicates that a distinction can be made between needs and need assessment. Existing definitions of needs can be categorized by the following perspectives: *type, level,* and *system.*[9] These categorizations are not mutually exclusive but overlap at different points. Need assessment, on the other hand, can be conceptualized as a process that includes a number of data collection steps and procedures for the purpose of documenting need, creating new programs, and modifying existing ones.

Bloom,[19] in this book, identifies several *types* of needs: recognized and unrecognized, met and unmet, private and public, and short-term and long-term. Nguyen, Attiksson, and Bottino[21] point out that needs exist on multiple *levels* and argue that definitions and strategies focusing on a single level, such as the individual or the community, are incomplete. Definitions can also be based on the perspectives of the client, service, and regulatory *systems.*[9,22] These correspond respectively to the service recipients, the service providers, and the laws, rules, and guidelines that regulate service provision.

In this volume, Nguyen, Attkisson, and Bottino[21] add further conceptual clarity to the assessment strategies, and their underlying assumptions, by classifying them according to *theoretical orientation.* According to these authors, each need assessment approach can be classified as rationalistic, as empirical, or as relativistic. Another contribution is their definition of unmet need which includes the following: (1) recognition of a problem, dysfunctional state, or undesirable social process; (2) judgment that satisfactory solutions are not accessible, adequate, or present; and (3) reallocation of existing resources or creation of new ones. Their conceptualization begins to identify the assessment steps necessary for responding to unmet needs.

Distinctions between need assessment and other evaluative research activities add further contributions. Nguyen and his associates[21] define need assessment as conceptually separate and operationally different from program evaluation. The former is an environmental monitoring system, designed to measure and make judgments about program relevance, adequacy, and appropriateness. Program evaluation, in contrast, is an internal monitoring system designed to assess program objective and mandates. Data are collected on such areas as service accessibility, comprehensiveness, and continuity and is used for program management, external accountability, and program planning.[23]

Similar contributions are made by Locke's distinction between need assessment and the epidemiologic approach.[20] The latter focuses primarily on "disease" prevention and control. In contrast, need assessment is primarily designed to assess service needs and to deploy agency resources for optimal recipient benefits. Although both use similar methods such as the survey technique, they can be distinguished by considering and contrasting their basic assumptions and purposes.

Recent developments have shed further light on definitional and conceptual issues. The field has begun to move beyond excessive reliance on administrative and organizational opinion and away from vague definitions that focus solely on the needs of the individual and/or community.[24] Needs and need assessment, as clearly pointed out in this volume and in this chapter, are complex. They are hierarchical, interconnected in both type and level, and have different theoretical origins. To disregard this complexity will lead only to a distorted and inaccurate picture of human needs. To assume that social scientists, at this time, would be able to agree on conceptualizations, definitions, and methods is also naive and premature.

In order to provide further coherence and integration, need assessors must clarify and relate such basic definitions and concepts as physical and mental illness, well being, and quality of life. These terms, as Turns and Newby[25] point out, too often remain vague and ill-defined thereby creating confusion and hindering communication. The transactional nature of needs and need assessment must also be recognized. Needs are clearly not static and to conceptualize them as so will only generate inaccurate data. Similarly, need assessment involves a dynamic process among a variety of constituents. Thus, conceptualizations and methods must incorporate this transactional dimension.

The field must be further anchored in scientific principles if progress is going to be made in defining need and in data collection and utility. According to Rychlak,[26] scientific theory serves four major functions. It is *descriptive*, that is, it allows for the explanation of phenomena. It is *delimiting*, organizing ideas into categories. It is generative, allowing the formulation of hypotheses. Finally, it is *integrating*, systematically incorporating data into a meaningful and consistent framework. Failure to apply scientific principles will lead to conceptual confusion and to unintegrated data. This lack of organization and inefficient use of information not only delimits each need assessment study but hinders the field as a whole.

In summary, changes are forthcoming in the area of need assessment. First, more attention will be paid to definitional and conceptual issues. Second, workers in the field will develop common and acceptable definitions of needs and need assessment. Third, the complex nature of needs will be recognized, and the theoretical underpinnings of various assessment strategies, such as the rationalistic, empirical, and relativistic, will be further articulated. Fourth, distinctions between need assessment and other activities such as program evaluation and epidemiologic studies will continue to be clarified. Finally, need assessment will further incorporate the scientific method as a way of improving its concepts and tools.

## METHODOLOGIC AND STRATEGY ISSUES

There currently exist a number of need assessment methods that provide different types of data that can be used for different purposes and vary considerably in their rigorousness. Each assessment approach can be analyzed according to (1) its theoretical and conceptual underpinnings, (2) its source of information, (3) reliability and validity of its data, (4) amount of "technical" expertise it requires, (5) amount of judgment required in translating its data into program operations, and (6) cost. Among the frequently used need assessment approaches discussed in this book are social indicators,[19] client utilization,[22] field survey,[27,28] nominal group,[29] and convergent assessment.[21] The methodologic and strategy issues will be discussed below in the context of these particular approaches.

The conceptual underpinnings of assessment methods vary considerably between those which are "atheoretical" and those with a clear rationale. Social indicators, for example, as Bloom[19] argues, are derived inductively rather than deductively; that is, the researcher uses some atheoretical procedure to select a set of social indicators from a pool of available data. On the other hand, client analysis, as presented by Scheff,[22] has a clear conceptual rationale. In between these polar extremes are a number of other methods. Survey approaches, for example, vary considerably depending on their purpose, method, and utility. The nominal group approach, derived from laboratory and field studies of group process and decision making, offers a clear rationale for processes but has no conceptual base for the nature of individuals, groups, organizations, or communities.

Need assessment strategies vary as to the source of their information. Social indicators and client utilization, for example, rely on secondary sources,[9] and the reliability of their data is variable providing opportunities for considerable error. Other approaches use first hand information. Surveys and the nominal group approach, for example, solicit data directly from the community at large, service recipients, and service providers. Since the data collection is under the control of the researcher, reliability can be checked, particularly with the survey method, and can even be improved.

Selection of assessment strategies has often been dictated by convenience, political expediency, and cost. Although these factors cannot be overlooked, one should not lose sight of the purpose of the assessment and the need to be methodologically rigorous. As Turns and Newby[25] point out in their chapter, need assessors and program people must be concerned with the reliability and validity of their strategies. There are, however, a number of factors that can jeopardize this rigorousness. Researchers, for example, use need assessment approaches idiosyncratically. They sometimes modify survey items to suit their own situation. Thus, few standard survey scales exist, hindering progress in the field since comparisons across studies and over time cannot readily be accomplished.

Uniformity within a particular need assessment approach should not be assumed. For example, social indicators can be developed theoretically, empirically, statistically, and clinically. Bloom[19] points out that broad constructs, such as quality of life, and even single social indicators, such as mental illness, may be constructed in a variety of ways. Standardization of need assessment approaches is needed before social scientists can determine the reliability, validity, and relative efficacy of each method. Such standardization would allow more effective comparisons between methods, more reliable longitudinal studies, and more accurate determination of program impacts.

Need assessment approaches vary in the "technical" expertise, that is, the amount of knowledge and experience, they require. Although some methods appear superficially simple, all can be complex depending on the purpose, scope, and type and amount of data collected. Client analysis, for example, can vary from the simple task of collecting service utilization data to the sophisticated process described by Scheff.[22] Conceptualizing need assessment as a planning function, she differentiates between two types of social planning, each of which is necessary but not sufficient for the development of rational policy and programs. Her seven-step, client-analysis method, which is more complex than the typical rates-under-treatment approach, requires a reasonable level of "technical" sophistication.

The more complicated the strategy used, the more the translation of data into program operations is hindered. Greater sophistication requires more "technical" expertise, and often experts lack the knowledge of, experience with, and sensitivity to programs and people that is necessary for a smooth transition from data to program operations. Greater complexity also requires more personnel and organizational structure to carry out the study. The possibilities of miscommunication among the assessors and between the assessors and program people are increased. Bigger and more complex need assessment strategies are not necessarily better. Care must be taken, therefore, not only in avoiding overly sophisticated need assessments, but also in curbing the tendency of social scientists to succumb to the temptation to gather excessive amounts of data.

Assessment strategies differ in the amount of judgment required to translate data into program operations. Social indicator data, in particular, because of its generality, must be judged more carefully than data from other strategies. Nominal group data has more variable requirements depending on how specifically the problem is posed to the group. Survey results vary considerably, but this approach can be designed so as to minimize the judgment process and to have programs follow reasonably directly from the data. Convergent assessments require first an integration of the diverse data, then a judgment as to the program implications. Thus, the nature of the need assessment strategy, in part, dictates the amount of judgment necessary for program planning.

Cost includes the total amount of program resources (money, supplies, staff time, etc.) needed to plan, carry out, and use a need assessment. It will depend on the scope and complexity of the assessment, as well as the size and complexity of the organization and its service programs. Social indicator approaches, usually characterized as "cheap," can be expensive if more sophisticated types are used. Surveys are usually characterized as "expensive" although a focused approach with volunteer staff can involve minimal cost. Because they use multiple approaches, convergent assessment methods will cost more than the others. Often overlooked is the amount of time required by the assessment project. Simple tasks such as gathering information from service recipients records, for example, can require a great deal of staff time.

Several writers in this volume have advocated using multiple need assessment approaches and convergent assessment models.[21,27] This approach, according to these individuals, has the advantage of providing a comprehensive picture of human service needs from multiple perspectives while compensating for individual strategy shortcomings.[9] It involves (1) integration of a wide range of data from multiple needs assessment strategies, (2) exploration of solutions to multiple health and human service problems, (3) an identification of types and levels of resources required for meeting identified needs, and (4) documentation of the priorities of needs and their solutions through the consensus of diverse constituents.[21]

There is a need in the field for greater methodologic specificity and diversity. The former is the detailed description, and implied standardization, of procedures and instruments. It allows the sharing of methods, findings, and conclusions from different studies to determine the appropriateness, effectiveness, and efficiency of their approaches. More laboratory and field work, such as that done by Delbecq and his associates[30-32] on the nominal group technique and by other investigators for social indicators, [33,34] is needed. Such research would allow (1) better articulation of the efficacy of the approaches, (2) further refinement of them, and (3) a clearer delineation of where single or multiple approaches are most appropriate.

Along with the further refinement and comparative studies of existing approaches, diversification is necessary. The field is too young to become complacent and set in using only existing methods in only conventional ways. More innovative applications of data to program planning are also needed. For example, Zautra,[28] in this volume, shows how a quality of life survey is useful for understanding the real-life problems of aged and Mexican-American groups and how this understanding can lead to the planning of mental health services for such individuals.

Efforts should also be made to incorporate existing knowledge from other social science disciplines. A substantive body of literature, for example, exists in the areas of community and ecologic psychology, organization process and development, and group process. This knowledge is rarely incorporated. Yet, it could be useful for both collecting data and utilizing data for program planning and development. Further linkages between theory and method are also needed. As pointed out earlier in this chapter, scientific theory serves a number of functions that are important for the further development of this field.

In the future, then, need assessors will need to (1) further articulate and clarify the theoretical and conceptual underpinnings of their strategies; (2) be more sensitive to the reliability and validity of the data gathered; (3) develop more standardized instruments that allow cross comparisons and longitudinal comparisons for the purpose of determining their appropriateness, efficiency, and effectiveness; (4) investigate the utility of multiple assessment approaches such as convergent analysis; and (5) maximize the fit between the theoretical or conceptual framework and the strategy used, particularly in light of the purposes and objectives of the need assessment.

## ISSUES IN APPLICATION, IMPLEMENTATION, AND UTILIZATION

Any need assessment project, as Murrell[35] points out, should provide information which, first of all, is reliable and valid and, second, is useful for program planning, development, and modification. Each factor, while necessary, is not sufficient in itself, yet a selected review of the literature finds that most authors focus on strategies. [10,13,17,36,37] Only recently have writers begun to attend to application, implementation, and utilization issues and the relevance of needs data to program decisions and for program managers. [12,14–16,38] One important problem in the use of data is the communication gaps among researchers, program people, and other relevant constituents. Guttentag[39] and Murrell, Aponte, and Lin,[40] for example, identify the array of decision makers and constituents, ranging from National Institute of Mental Health staff to citizen groups, who have a stake in need assessment. The different values, goals, and agendas of each constituent create obstacles in utilizing data.

As Murrell[14] points out, need assessors tend to focus on data while program managers are concerned with the organizational consequences of their decisions. He argues that the bigger the gap between the kind of information needed by managers and that supplied by researchers, the lower the probability of the data being used. To increase usage, need assessors must tailor their data to correspond to the questions raised by managers. Murrell[35,38] goes on to identify eight steps for converting data into program operations that are likely to maximize data utilization. A particularly important step is determining the sponsor's "feared risks" prior to carrying out the assessment. Equally important is relating this tolerance to the assessment methods. Each technique has the potential of either minimizing or maximizing organization risks and thus impacting on the utilization of collected data.

Other mechanisms have been proposed to narrow the gap

between data and program people. Sundel, in this book and elsewhere[41,42] identifies a number of steps that researchers can take within an organization to maximize data utilization. Davis[43] even recommends the creation of an "intermediary advocate" who would bridge the chasm between data and planning. Such an individual would function as a consultant to both research and program people. The present gaps separating people who collect data from program administrators, directors, and service providers will continue to narrow. Need assessors are becoming more sensitive and responsive to programs, their operations, and the complexities of program planning. Program people are beginning to understand data and to feel comfortable working with it. Each is beginning to understand the language of the other.

Once need assessors and program people are talking to and understanding one another, a critical next step is the agreement of all interested parties on the implications for program planning and development. The issue of how data is translated into program operations is addressed by Guttentag's Multi-Attribute Utilities and Bayesian Statistical Method (MAUT-Bayesian Model).[39] This model has a number of complex steps, but basically it involves decision makers in the process of assigning priorities and thus gives them a stake in the utilization of data. Such models will begin to identify the necessary processes in maximizing the use of need assessment data.

Clarification of the necessary steps between data collection and the application, implementation, and utilization of findings in program operations is needed. The key people in this process and the roles that each play also have to be further identified. Unless such action is taken, need assessments will have the same fate as many evaluation studies and will go unused to the detriment of service providers and service recipients.[44] Distinctions also have to be made among application, implementation, and utilization. Application can be conceptualized as the initial step in using data and entails at least the reading of a report or the discussion of findings. Implementation is the next logical step— working with the data and planning how to use it. Utilization involves the actual use of data for program development or modification.

Thus, need assessors in their future application, implementation, and utilization of data should: (1) recognize and identify the complexities of using data for program planning, (2) determine and be sensitive to the organization's "risk-tolerance," (3) incorporate steps that will narrow the gap between research and program people, (4) guide procedures into the assessment process to ensure the usage of collected data in creating new programs and improving existing ones, and (5) research the efficacy of different strategies to ensure that data are eventually used in planning, not collecting dust on administrators' shelves.

## CONCLUSIONS

The field of need assessment is a young and burgeoning area although some of the ideas and data gathering strategies used are not new.[40] Progress has been made in conceptualization, methodology, and utilization, but further work is clearly called for. A balance is needed between the research and practical aspects of assessment. Too much attention on methodologic rigorousness and not enough on the organizational and social contexts, for example, may lead to highly reliable and valid data that goes unused. Thus, research into the "pure" and "applied" aspects of need assessment is also necessary.

Some individuals suggest that the basic assumptions underlying need assessment should be reexamined. Turns and Newby,[25] for example, question whether measuring health status necessarily leads to better service delivery. They argue that entry into treatment is often influenced by factors other than the presence of physical or mental illness. Distance, economics, attitudes, and administrative policies will often dictate who does or does not receive services. It is thus naive to think that measurement of needs translates directly into program objectives. Turns and Newby also point out that it is presumptuous to believe that one can treat all identified illnesses or meet all community needs. Such a belief will only lead to frustrated expectations.

Despite these potential pitfalls and the issues and problems pointed out earlier, the field of need assessment will continue to grow. The impetus for this change will be those factors pointed out at the beginning of this book by Murrell, Aponte, and Lin[40] and of this chapter: legislative mandates, emphasis on rational planning and accountability, and the stress on meeting recipient needs. Legislative mandates will become even more important as public servants at federal, state, and local levels become more concerned with tax revenues and as more demands are made on limited amounts of money. Service programs, because of these limited resources, will be forced to justify the existence of their programs as they compete for funds.

Need assessment will continue to become more sophisticated and to be applied beyond the health and human service fields. Needs will no longer be defined solely in terms of a method, and divergent conceptualizations and strategies will become more important. The assessment process will receive more attention, particularly that aspect dealing with the application, implementation, and utilization of data for program planning and development.[38,45] Additional attention will have to be paid to the social and political climate[6] because data in itself has little significance and utility unless it is congruent with these realities. It can, however, change them if the critical elements affecting the social context can be identified.

Convergent conceptual schemes will be further developed and play an important role.[21] However, it should not be assumed that convergent analysis is a panacea for definitional, conceptual, and methodologic problems. Using a number of unreliable methods, for example, still yields unreliable data. This approach needs further developing and empirical testing. Development of other models is also important for conceptual and methodologic advances, and behavioral and social scientists and program people should be involved in this process.

Need assessors will have to be open to the growing contributions of other disciplines. Additional laboratory and field studies, where one technique is pitted against another, will be needed, particularly as new methods are added. Such studies will facilitate the determination of the reliability, validity, and efficacy of the various approaches. The communication and exchange of ideas, concepts, and methodologies will thus become more important as individuals from other disciplines become increasingly involved. The development of common and clearly understood vocabularies will be critical.

The focus will have to shift away from people who are already physically or psychologically impaired and toward those who may be at psychological and physical risk. As Dohrenwend[46] suggests in this volume, the investigation of mental stressors that induce disorders in vulnerable individuals is of critical importance. Social stressors, described as stressful life events, are one way of identifying those at risk. Interventions designed and planned for these high-risk individuals have potentially greater impact on the community and society than programs solely designed to repair existing psychological, physical, and social damage.

This volume represents one of the most comprehensive works to date in the field of need assessment in health and human services. It is not intended to be a "how-to" manual; several excellent ones already exist.[13,15,16,30] Rather, its purpose is to describe the "state of the art" and identify the substantive issues at definitional, conceptual, methodologic, and utilization levels. While it is clear that much work remains to be done, the progress of the past decade indicates that the field will continue to grow and develop at a healthy pace to the benefit of service providers and recipients alike.

## Notes

1. Kimmel, W. A. *Needs assessment: A critical perspective.* Washington, D.C.: Department of Health, Education and Welfare, Office of the Assistant Secretary for Planning and Evaluation, 1977.

2. Zangwill, B. *A compendium of laws and regulations requiring needs assessment.* Washington, D.C.: Department of Health, Education and Welfare, Office of the Assistant Secretary for Planning and Evaluation, 1977.

3. Hapenney, S. The impact of P.L. 93-641, the National Health Planning and Resources Development Act, upon health and mental health programming, *Journal of Evaluation and Program Planning,* 1978, *1,* 79–81.

4. Milstein, A. Anticipating the impact of Public Law 93–641 on mental health services. *American Journal of Psychiatry,* 1976, *33,* 710–712.

5.  Mondale, W. Social accounting, evaluation and the future of the human services. *Evaluation,* 1972, *1,* 29–34.

6.  Peterson, R. L. Social mandates and Federal legislation: Implications for health planning. In R. A. Bell, M. Sundel, J. F. Aponte, & S. A. Murrell (Eds.), *Need Assessment in Health and Human Services: Proceedings of the Louisville National Conference.* Louisville, 1976.

7.  Schwab, J. J. (See Chapter 1, this volume).

8.  Ibid., 16.

9.  Aponte, J. F. A need in search of a theory and an approach. *Journal of Community Psychology,* 1978, *6,* 42–44.

10. Bloom, B. L. The assessment of community structure and community needs. In B. L. Bloom, *Community mental health: A general introduction.* Monterey, Calif.: Brooks/Cole, 1977.

11. Blum, H. L. *Planning for health: Development and application of social change theory.* New York: Human Sciences Press, 1974.

12. Center for Social Research and Development. *An analysis and synthesis of needs assessment research in the field of human services.* Denver: Denver Research Institute, 1974.

13. Hargreaves, W. A., Attkisson, C. C., Siegal, L. M., McIntyre, M. H., & Sorensen, J. E. (Eds.). *Resource materials for community mental health program evaluation, Part III: Needs assessment and planning.* Washington, D.C.: National Institute of Mental Health, 1974.

14. Murrell, S. A. Utilization of needs assessment for community decision-making. *American Journal of Community Psychology,* 1977, *5,* 461–468.

15. Warheit, G. J., Bell, R. A., & Schwab, J. J. *Planning for change: Needs assessment approaches.* Rockville, Md.: National Institute of Mental Health, 1974.

16. Warheit, G. J., Bell, R. A., & Schwab, J. J. *Needs assessment approaches: Concepts and methods.* Rockville, Md.: National Institute of Mental Health, 1977.

17. Siegel, L. M., Attkisson, C. C., & Carson, L. G. Need identification and program planning in the community context. In C. C. Attkisson, W. A. Hargreaves, M. J. Horowitz, & J. E. Sorensen (Eds.), *Evaluation of human service programs.* New York: Academic Press, 1978.

18.  Broskowski, A. (See Chapter 4, this volume).

19.  Bloom, B. L. (See Chapter 8, this volume).

20.  Locke, B. Z. (See Chapter 3, this volume).

21.  Nguyen, T. D., Attkisson, C. C., & Bottino, M. J. (See Chapter 5, this volume).

22.  Scheff, J. (See Chapter 9, this volume).

23.  Attkisson, C. C., & Broskowski, A. Evaluation and the emerging human service concept. In C. C. Attkisson, W. A. Hargreaves, M. J. Horowitz, & J. E. Sorensen (Eds.), *Evaluation of human service programs.* New York: Academic Press, 1978.

24.  Aponte, J. F. Implications for the future of need assessment. In R. A. Bell, M. Sundel, J. F. Aponte, & S. A. Murrell (Eds.), *Need assessment in health and human services: Proceedings of the Louisville National Conference.* Louisville, 1976.

25.  Turns, D. M. & Newby, L. G. (See Chapter 6, this volume).

26.  Rychlak, J. F. *A philosophy of science for personality theory.* Boston: Houghton Mifflin, 1968.

27.  Warheit, G. J., & Bell, R. A. (See Chapter 10, this volume).

28.  Zautra, A., Goodhart, D., & Kochanowicz, N. (See Chapter 11, this volume).

29.  Delbecq, A. L. (See Chapter 12, this volume).

30.  Delbecq, A. L., Van de Ven, A. J., & Gustafson, D. H. *Group techniques for program planning: A guide to Nominal Group and Delphi processes.* Glenview, Ill.: Scott, Foresman, 1975.

31.  Van de Ven, A. H., & Delbecq, A. L. Nominal vs. interacting group processes for committee decision-making effectiveness. *Academy of Management Journal,* 1971, *14,* 204–211.

32.  Van de Ven, A. H., & Delbecq, A. L. The effectiveness of Nominal, Delphi, and interacting group decision-making processes. *Academy of Management Journal,* 1974, *17,* 605–621.

33.  Buhl, J. M., Warheit, G. J., & Bell, R. A. The key informant approach to community needs assessment: A case study. *Evaluation and Program Planning,* 1978, *1,* 239–247.

34.  Warheit, G. J. Buhl, J. M., & Bell, R. A. A critique of social indica-

tors analysis and key informants surveys as needs assessment methods. *Evaluation and Program Planning*, 1978, *1*, 23–30.

35. Murrell, S. A. (See Chapter 15, this volume).

36. Bell, R. A., Warheit, G. J., & Schwab, J. J. Need assessment: A strategy for structuring change. In R. D. Coursey, G. A. Specter, S. A. Murrell, & B. Hunt, (Eds.), *Program evaluation for mental health: Methods, strategies, participants.* New York: Grune & Stratton, 1976.

37. Bell, R. A., Nguyen, T. D., Warheit, G. J., & Buhl, J. M. Service utilization, social indicator, and citizen survey approaches to human service need assessment. In C. C. Attkisson, W. A. Hargreaves, M. J. Horowitz, & J. E. Sorensen (Eds.), *Evaluation of human service programs.* New York: Academic Press, 1978.

38. Murrell, S. A. Eight process steps for converting need assessment data into program operations. In R. A. Bell, M. Sundel, J. F. Aponte, & S. A. Murrell (Eds.), *Need assessment in health and human services: Proceedings of the Louisville National Conference.* Louisville, 1976.

39. Guttentag, M. (See Chapter 13, this volume).

40. Murrell, S. A., Aponte, J. F., & Lin, E. (See Introduction, this volume).

41. Sundel, M. (See Chapter 14, this volume).

42. Morrison, B. J., & Sundel, M. Development of a community assessment strategy for program evaluation in a comprehensive human service delivery system. In J. Zusman & C. Wurster (Eds.), *Program evaluation: Alcohol, drug abuse, and mental health services.* Lexington, Mass.: D.C. Heath, 1975.

43. Davis, S. *Needs assessment as a developmental process: The case for an intermediary advocate.* Chapel Hill: University of North Carolina, 1974.

44. Weiss, C. *Evaluating action programs.* Boston: Allyn & Bacon, 1972.

45. Aponte, J. F. *The process of mental health needs assessment and program planning.* Louisville, Kentucky: Department of Psychology, University of Louisville, 1975.

46. Dohrenwend, B. S. (See Chapter 7, this volume).

*Chapter 18*

# AN ANNOTATED BIBLIOGRAPHY IN NEED ASSESSMENT IN HEALTH AND HUMAN SERVICES

*Joseph F. Aponte,*
*Pamela M. Leone,*
*Roger A. Bell*

## INTRODUCTION

The purpose of this annotated bibliography is to provide a selected overview of readings in need assessment in health and human services. It is intended to provide the novice with sufficient material to obtain a broad view of the current state of need assessment activities. There are also a number of readings identified in each section that allow the more serious reader to acquire depth in a given area.

Because of the large number of publications in the field, no attempt was made to cover these topics exhaustively nor to evaluate them qualitatively. For example, over 1,000 social indicators references are listed alone by Wilcox et al. (1972). Similarly, a number of articles, monographs, and working papers are published by organizations such as the National Institute of Mental Health and the Institute for Social Research, University of Michigan, that are better solicited directly.

This chapter is divided into six sections. The first contains overviews and comprehensive readings. These works usually extend beyond mental health to include health and human services.

Section two includes references related to either the planning of a need assessment or the planning of services and programs. The third section, need assessment strategies, includes citations for rates-under-treatment (service utilization), social indicators, nominal group and delphi technique, survey, and other approaches.

Section four deals with the utilization and application of collected data. The fifth section covers examples of need assessment studies, including pilot and demonstration projects. Although there are a large number of studies that have been conducted, very few have been published; most of them are either in-house publications or are not widely distributed. Finally, the last section lists related readings that are of potential utility to individuals interested in need assessment in health and human services.

## OVERVIEWS AND COMPREHENSIVE READINGS

Aponte, J. F. A need in search of a theory and an approach. *Journal of Community Psychology*, 1978, *6*, 42–44.

Major points in this article are drawn from the proceedings of the First National Conference on Need Assessment in Health and Human Services. Theoretical and conceptual issues are identified. Frequently used need assessment methodologies such as social indicators, client utilization, survey, nominal group, and convergent assessment approaches are also discussed. Finally, the need to integrate theory and assessment approaches is identified in order to have effective decision making, program planning, knowledge building, and theory testing.

Bell R. A., & Mellan, W. *Southern health and family studies (Vol. I). An assessment of needs: An epidemiologic survey.* Gainesville, Fla.: Florida Mental Health Evaluation Consortium, 1974.

Briefly described in this monograph is a comprehensive evaluation model that includes: (1) evaluation activities, including descriptive assessments of needs, comparative analysis, outcome appraisal, and community impact studies; (2) systems of intervention, such as outpatient and emergency services; and (3) purposes, including research, treatment, management information, and comprehensive planning information. A general description of instruments used to identify social psychiatric impairment is also included in the monograph.

Bell, R. A., Sundel, M., Aponte, J. F., & Murrell, S. A. (Eds.). Need assessment in health and human services: Proceedings of the Louisville National Conference. Louisville, Kentucky, 1976. A comprehensive set of readings in health and human services based on the First National Conference on Need Assessment in Health and Human Services held in Louisville, Kentucky in 1976, this volume consists of presentations from experts in a variety of fields and disciplines. Among the topics included are: (1) theoretical issues; (2) planning a need assessment; (3) need assessment strategies, including social indicators, client analysis, survey, nominal group, and convergent assessment approaches; and (4) utilization and application of data to the modification and planning of service programs.

Bell, R. A., Nguyen, T. D., Warheit, G. J., & Buhl, J. M. Service utilization, social indicator, and citizen survey approaches to human service need assessment. In C. C. Attkisson, W. A. Hargreaves, M. J. Horowitz, & J. E. Sorensen (Eds.), *Evaluation of human service programs*. New York: Academic Press, 1978, pp. 253–300.
This chapter presents a detailed examination of the more complex need assessment approaches in terms of their designs, costs, advantages, and disadvantages. The discussion includes an overview of need assessment, specification of data sources and types of data, and detailed descriptions of data gathering and analysis, for example, instrument development and coding procedures. Also included are suggestions for the presentations of findings. Each approach is well-illustrated by data from actual need assessment studies.

Bell, R. A., Warheit, G. J., & Schwab, J. J. Need assessment: A strategy for structuring change. In R. D. Coursey, G. A. Specter, S. A. Murrell, & B. Hunt. *Program evaluation for mental health: Methods, strategies, participants*. New York: Grune and Stratton, 1976, pp. 67–76.
A brief and concise overview of need assessment is provided

in this chapter. A working definition of need assessment is articulated as are brief descriptions of available need assessment approaches, including: (1) key informant, (2) community forums, (3) rates-under-treatment, (4) social indicators, and (5) surveys. The advantages and disadvantages of each are identified. The authors recommend that, when possible, a combination or series of studies be used to assess needs.

Bloom, B. L. The assessment of community structure and community needs. In B. L. Bloom (Ed.), *Community mental health: A general introduction.* Monterey, Calif.: Brooks/Cole, 1977, pp. 173–205.

Dr. Bloom draws a parallel between the assessment of community characteristics and the assessment of individual characteristics. In this chapter, a brief discussion of various concepts of community is followed by a detailed discussion of social indicators, including: (1) a brief history and definition of social indicators, (2) selection of social indicators, and (3) problems with social indicators. The utilization of community-subarea analyses is discussed followed by a section on the utilization of other strategies for assessing community needs, such as expert assessment of needs and the assessment of community opinion.

Hagedorn, H. J., Beck, K. J., Neubert, S. F., & Werlin, S. H. *A working manual of simple program evaluation techniques for community mental health centers.* Rockville, Md.: National Institute of Mental Health, 1976.

The purpose of this manual is to present in a convenient form a variety of program evaluation techniques and approaches. Included in the volume are basic concepts, reviews of several basic evaluation tools, technical topics in program evaluation, and citizen review of community mental health centers. Of particular interest is chapter four which discusses a variety of commonly used need assessment approaches.

Hargreaves, W. A., Attkisson, C. C., Siegal, L. M., McIntyre, M. H., & Sorenson, J. E. (Eds.). *Resource materials for community mental health program evaluation. Part III: Needs assessment and planning.* Rockville, Md.: National Institute of Mental Health, 1974.

Four presentations illustrate a variety of approaches in need assessment, and each focuses on a particular aspect of the process. The chapter on "Mental Health Needs Assessment: Strategies and Techniques" provides a concise overview of the field. Several strategies and techniques are reviewed in detail; social area analysis and a group process model are discussed separately. In addition, the procedures of goal analysis are outlined in an abstract.

Lemkau, P. Assessing a community's need for mental health services. *Hospital and Community Psychiatry,* 1967, *18,* 13–18.

This paper presents a general overview of need assessment ranging from historical background to particular problems of different approaches. Hospital statistics, psychiatric registers, and surveys are discussed as data sources. However, definitional issues are continually emphasized and revolve around the question "who needs what?" The implications for future directions are discussed by the author.

Mondale, W. Social accounting, evaluation and the future of the human services. *Evaluation,* 1972, *1,* 29–34.

This essay presents a rationale for evaluating human services from the perspective of a former United States Senator who had been active in generating relevant legislation. Developing an information system that can enhance goal setting and prioritization is discussed, and several approaches to evaluation are highlighted. Also, key government agencies and offices are frequently cited throughout the text as they relate to the specific problem being examined.

Siegel, L. M., Attkisson, C. C., & Carson, L. G. Need identification and program planning in the community context. In C. C. Attkisson, W. A. Hargreaves, M. J. Horowitz, & J. E. Sorensen (Eds.), *Evaluation of human service programs.* New York: Academic Press, 1978, pp. 215–252.

A well-developed rationale for need identification and assessment is presented in this chapter. It begins with basic definitions and arguments concerning justification for such studies. Need assessment goals are directly related to program development and evaluation, and their interface is discussed. However, the major portion of the chapter offers a comprehensive methodology overview that continually emphasizes coordination and integration of services, rationalization of planning, and consumer-professional cooperation as goal components inherent in need identification and assessment.

Varenais, K. *Needs assessment: An exploratory critique.* Washington, D. C.: Department of Health, Education, and Welfare, 1977.

This paper examines the uses and definitions of "need assessment" and the methodologies used to assess needs by reviewing books, manuals, journal articles, and legislation in the area. Several potential interpretations of "need assessment" are cited, and a critique of its potential utility is offered. An annotated bibliography of "need assessment" literature is also included.

Warheit, G. J., Bell, R. A., & Schwab, J. J. *Needs assessment approaches: Concepts and methods.* Rockville, Md.: National Institute of Mental Health, 1977.

The updated edition of an earlier monograph (Warheit, Bell, & Schwab, 1974), this manual is designed to serve as a resource for those involved in conducting need assessment studies in community settings. Among the material included are the following: (1) descriptions of five need assessment approaches, (2) activity checklists, (3) work sheets, and (4) data collection instruments and other research aids. Such materials have potential utility to individuals in community mental health centers and other human service settings.

Zangwill, B. *A compendium of laws and regulations requiring needs assessment.* Washington, D. C.: Department of Health, Education, and Welfare, 1977.

Included in this study is an identification of Department of Health, Education, and Welfare programs requiring need assessment in their statutes or regulations. Relevant excerpts from these statutes and regulations are provided, as well as an analysis of these requirements. Among the factors included are: (1) clarity of the need assessment requirement, (2) document in which need assessment is contained, (3) who conducts the need assessment, and (4) specification of the need assessment technique and its frequency.

## II. NEED ASSESSMENT AND PLANNING

Babigian, H. M. The role of epidemiology and mental health care statistics in the planning of mental health centers. In A. Beigel & A. I. Levenson (Eds.), *The community mental health centers: Strategies and programs.* New York: Basic Books, 1973, pp. 32–47.

After a brief introduction, the author focuses on the utilization of data from the psychiatric register for planning mental health services in Monroe County, New York. The psychiatric case register is discussed in terms of providing information on patient load and utilization of facilities. The data are then applied in projecting the number of beds and demand for outpatient and emergency services as related to the development of new mental health centers.

Blum, H. L. *Planning for health: Development and application of social change theory.* New York: Human Sciences Press, 1974.

Dr. Blum articulates a comprehensive perspective on planning based on the development and application of social change theory. After discussing the systems approach to health care, he presents detailed analyses of the environment for planning, the determination of desired improvements, achievement of improvements, and measurement of the obtained improvements. The role of assessment and evaluation strategies in effective planning is highlighted.

Gwen, A. Uses of data in planning community psychiatric services. *American Journal of Public Health,* 1965, *55,* 1925–1935.

A general approach for using data in planning community psychiatric services is proposed by the author. Included in this approach are the following: (1) characterization of the relevant target population, (2) measurement of the movement of the population through the total care system, (3) use of census control methods, (4) resource allocation for maximum effectiveness, and (5) maximum use of modern instrumentation and computers. The author also suggests the unification of different systems to provide a common statistical base of various kinds of services.

Hapenney, S. The impact of P.L. 93–641, the National Health Planning and Resources Development Act, upon health and mental health programming. *Journal of Evaluation and Program Planning*, 1978, *1*, 79–81.

This paper reviews the P.L. 93–641 in terms of its development, its interpretation, and its potential impact on community health care programs. The narrative is directed toward assisting local health care providers in relating with the health systems agencies established by the law. In general, according to the author, new health planning will require cooperative efforts from diverse groups and constituents, such as consumers and service providers.

Milstein, A. Anticipating the impact of Public Law 93–641 on mental health services. *American Journal of Psychiatry*, 1976, *33*, 710–712.

Interviews with mental health care providers, planners, and citizen representatives provide the basis for this article. The author assesses the law's potential ramifications in terms of six major issues: joint planning of health services, the integration of health systems agencies with existing mechanisms, evaluation, consumer input, technical expertise, and regional planning. The emphasis is on enlightening health planning professionals about the benefits and plausible difficulties that can be anticipated.

Palmiere, D. Problems in local community planning of mental illness facilities and services. *American Journal of Public Health*, 1965, *55*, 561–569.

Using mental illness as a "case" example, the author discusses some of the major factors in service delivery systems and community organizations that affect the planning process. Five specific problem areas are highlighted: (1) inadequate understanding of mental illness, (2) changing patterns of services and facilities, (3) organization and financing of services, (4) selected pressures on local communities, and (5) the process of local community planning.

Schulberg, H. C., & Wechsler, H. The uses and misuses of data in assessing mental health needs. *Community Mental Health Journal,* 1967, *3*, 389–395.

The authors focus upon the need assessment procedures stipulated by the 1964 Federal Regulations for the Community Mental Health Centers Act. The assumptions underlying these procedures are identified, and their significance for planners is discussed. There are inherent theoretical difficulties and methodologic limitations in these regulations. However, the authors feel that these regulations will ultimately broaden the planners' definition of community need.

Weiss, A. T. Consumer model of assessing community mental health needs. *Exchange,* 1973, *7*, 14–16.

This paper presents a specific application of a consumer model in order to gain information about priorities of need categorized by target problem, age group, and geographic area. Five groups surveyed include mental health agencies, referral agencies, high-risk individuals (service users), civic groups, and the community-at-large (random sample). The simplicity of the model is emphasized as the data is analyzed, and the specific recommendations are illustrated.

## III. Need Assessment Strategies

### A. Rates-Under-Treatment (Service and Client Utilization)

Berger, D. G., & Gardner, E. A. Use of community surveys in mental health planning. *American Journal of Public Health,* 1971, *61*, 110–118.

The title of this paper is somewhat misleading. The study described involved comparing utilization rates from two different time points in order to assess the impact of establishing a community mental health center in an urban disadvantaged community. Arguments are advanced for going beyond utilization rates in planning mental health services and in garnering public support for such programs in the community.

Fennell, E. G., Schwab, J. J., Warheit, G. J., Lund, D. A., Josephson, S., & Spencer, M. *Evaluating Alachua County's mental health needs and services: Rates-under-treatment.* Gainesville, Fla.: Departments of Psychiatry and Sociology, University of Florida, 1973.

As one part of a five-year research program designed to investigate the mental health needs and services in a southern county, prevailing patterns of care and types of available treatment were surveyed. Sociodemographic characteristics of cases treated by the services examined are reported in this paper. In addition, data is reported on: (1) sources and reasons for referral, (2) history of previous medical or psychiatric hospitalization, (3) patient disposition, (4) referral system within the county, and (5) comparisons of clients of four agencies with county residents.

Levy, B., & Bell, R. A. *Aftercare service needs in a metropolitan area: An assessment of client utilization.* A paper presented at the Second National Conference on Need Assessment in Health and Human Services. University of Louisville, Louisville, Kentucky, 1978.

This study reports on the following types of data for an aftercare facility located in a metropolitan area: (1) basic demographic information; (2) diagnosis, treatment, medication, and hospitalization; (3) referral services, attendance, and program information; and (4) presenting problem, goals, and attainment of these goals. The implications for future investigations for this setting are pointed out by the authors.

Reiner, J. S., Reimer, E., & Reiner, T. A. Client analysis and the planning of public programs. *Journal of the American Institute of Planners,* 1963, *20,* 270–282.

A rationale is provided for the use of client analysis, and ten steps outlining the progression of this approach are presented. The analysis encompasses needs, eligibility, service rendered, and client satisfaction while the discussion addresses issues ranging from standards of service to legislative input. A hypothetical example is used to illustrate the application of client analysis, and recommendations are offered based on the merits of this approach.

B. *Social Indicators*

Agocs, C. Social indicators. Selected readings. *The Annals of the American Academy of Political and Social Sciences*, 1970, *388*, 127–132.

Included in these selected readings are: (1) relevant books, (2) chapters from books, (3) journal articles, (4) public statements by government officials, and (5) presentations at professional meetings. Although limited in scope, these readings are potentially useful in developing a basic background in the area of social indicators. Some of the references in the article are annotated by the author.

Bauer, R. (Ed.). *Social indicators.* Cambridge, Mass.: MIT Press, 1966.

This volume contains chapters by distinguished authors in the area of social indicators. Although written in anticipation of the secondary effects of the space program, the material in this book has general implications for monitoring and anticipating the general state of society. Particular attention is directed toward the sections written by Albert Biderman, "Social Indicators and Goals," and Bertram Gross, "The State of the Nation: Social Systems Accounting."

Beal, G. M., Brocks, R. M., Wilcox, L. D., and Klonglan, G. E. *Social indicators: Bibliography I.* Ames, Iowa: Iowa State University, 1971.

The extensive bibliography is prefaced by a review of selected writings on social indicators and a discussion of the project at Iowa State University. The authors also describe the procedures used for reviewing the literature and for obtaining the materials included in this bibliography.

Bell, W. Social areas: Typology of neighborhoods. In M. Sussman (Ed.), *Community structure and analysis.* New York: Cromwell, 1959, 61–92.

This essay presents social area analysis as a method for classifying and describing different communities. The use of economic, family, and ethnic characteristics as they appear in census tract data is discussed both theoretically and empirically. Major contributors and important studies are reviewed, and computations for the indices are included. The author summarizes by outlining the most effective applications of this typology and by suggesting future possibilities.

Bloom, B. L. A census tract analysis of socially deviant behaviors. *Multivariate Behavioral Research*, 1966, *1*, 307–320.

Characteristics of census tracts and measures of social equilibrium are described, and the intercorrelation of social equilibrium across tracts is examined for a western city of approximately 120,000. The discussion focuses upon the selection of census tract demographic and environmental characteristics that are associated with individual types of social behavioral deviation. The data analysis is illustrated in several tables. Methodologic problems are noted, and concluding remarks explore the difficulties with inferring causal relationships.

Bloom, B. L. An ecological analysis of psychiatric hospitalizations. *Multivariate Behavioral Research*, 1968, *3*, 423–463.

This article is based on a study of census tract data for Pueblo, Colorado. The differential relationships between first admission rates and a cluster analysis of the social structure are explored. Four well-defined clusters include socioeconomic affluence, young marrieds, social isolation, and social disequilibrium. Dr. Bloom also offers comparisons with other ecologic analyses. The major implications focus on the potential for the development of preventive strategies and the continued refinement of social etiology.

Davis, S. *Needs assessment as a developmental process: The case for an intermediary advocate.* Chapel Hill: University of North Carolina, 1974.

This extensive paper surveys community mental health planning; discusses in detail three sources of social information—psychiatric epidemiology, social indicators, U.S. Census; and presents a thorough description of small area analysis. The author argues for structuring need assessment activity developmentally aligned with the norms of program consultation. Consultation is presented as bridging the chasm between available data and social planning needs.

Faris, R. E. L., & Dunham, H. W. *Mental disorders in urban areas: An ecological study of schizophrenia and other psychoses.* New York: Hafner, 1961.

This book is a reprint of the 1939 pioneer study on the social aspects of mental disorder. The data illuminates the association of different types of psychoses with specific community characteristics. The well-illustrated text discusses patterns of distribution for various types of psychoses, including those related to alcohol, drugs, and old age, in Chicago and Providence. Theoretical assumptions about the interplay of constitutional, psychological, and sociological factors in mental disorders are explored in depth.

Goldsmith, H. F., & Unger, E. L. *Mental health demographic profile for Prince George's County.* Rockville, Md.: National Institute of Mental Health, 1973.

This study provides a model for the delineation of meaningful social areas and for inferences about the needs of the resident populations of each area. The components of social rank and life-style dimensions are illustrated in detail. Other indicators such as ethnicity and homogeneity are also included in this example of a small area data profile system.

Goldsmith, H. F., & Unger, E. L. Area economic status, area social status, and area family life cycle in suburban communities. *Journal of Community Psychology,* 1975, *3,* 231–238.

The differential relationship of economic status and social area status with family life cycles is explored in order to demonstrate that area socioeconomic status should not be treated as a unidimensional variable. Prince George's County data is analyzed and used to substantiate the argument for retaining the three aforementioned measures as independent dimensions.

Goldsmith, H. F., Rosen, B. M., Shambaugh, J. P., Stockwell, E. G., & Windle, C. D. *Demographic norms for metropolitan, nonmetropolitan and rural counties.* Rockville, Md.: National Institute of Mental Health, 1975.

The major goal of this paper is to illustrate how different social areas can be compared using the Mental Health Demographic Profile System. Selected percentile values for 130 social indicators are presented, thus providing a simple basis for classifying and ranking specific areas according to their particular characteristics. The authors argue that the evaluative classification offers an empirically-based rationale for the planning and allocation of services.

Hawley, A. H., & Duncan, O. Social area analysis: A critical appraisal. *Land Economics,* 1957, *33,* 337–345.

The authors raise major questions related to the use of social area analysis. Their concerns revolve around the definition of "social area," the nature of empirical identification, and the theoretical justification for the methodology. They discuss several approaches—the empirical, the analogical, the stratification theory, and the functional system—and note the weaknesses of each one. It is suggested that the serious problems illustrated be remedied before any technique is recognized as making valuable contributions.

Kanno, C. K. *Eleven indices: An aid in reviewing state and local mental health and hospital programs.* Washington, D.C.: The Joint Information Service, 1971.

This revision of *Fifteen Indices* (1957) includes six new indices and has deleted ten from the previous publication. Each index is discussed and illustrated in tabular form for all states. Summary graphs for each state on all eleven indices complete the presentation. These indices have potential utility in the planning of local and state mental health and hospital programs.

Kay, F. D. Applications of social area analysis to program planning and evaluation. *Journal of Evaluation and Program Planning,* 1978, *1,* 65–78.

Social area analysis as a research technique is discussed in detail using specific examples that are graphically well-illustrated. One application focuses on demographic variables, and the other examines the use of social area analysis for developing meaningful descriptors of a hospital's community. Also the article offers several suggestions for those endeavoring to develop similar research approaches.

Land, K. C. On the definition of social indicators. *The American Sociologist*, 1971, *6*, 322–325.

This paper addresses critical evaluations of the use of social indicators, and, in particular, responds to the arguments set forth by Sheldon and Freeman in "Notes on social indicators: Promises and potential" (*Policy Sciences*, 1970, *1*, 97–111). The author proposes a definitional criterion based on social indicators as input or output variables in a social systems model and emphasizes the need for refining these models.

Land, K. C. Social indicator models: An overview. In K. C. Land, & S. Spilerman (Eds.), *Social indicator models*. New York: Russell Sage Foundation, 1974.

Three rationales for social indicators are surveyed in depth—social policy, social change, and social reporting, and their common characteristics are recognized. Social indicators are defined and classified according to type and model. However, the major presentation is a paradigm for social indicator models that examines their substantive contents and their contribution to the analysis of social change.

Miller, F. T., Aponte, J. F., Bentz, W. K., Edgerton, W. J., & Hollister, H. G. *Experiences in rural mental health: Measuring and monitoring stress in communities*. Chapel Hill: University of North Carolina Press, 1974.

Representing one of a series of booklets in *Experiences in rural mental health*, this work deals with the measuring and monitoring of stress in communities. The activities of this federally funded project included: (1) monitoring of public events; (2) monitoring of private events, such as individual perceptions and responses to stress; and (3) the development of single and multiple variable indices of stress. The exploratory use of social area analysis for identifying mental health needs is also discussed.

Mustain, R. D., & See, J. J. Indicators of mental health needs: An empirical and pragmatic evaluation. *Journal of Health and Social Behavior*, 1973, *14*, 23–27.

Correlational analyses are used in this study to assess the similarities between mental health need priority systems for six southern states and priority systems developed using a simplified scheme of mental health indicators. The results indicate a significant correlation. The authors suggest that time and effort not be spent in constructing elaborate priority systems when simpler strategies are available.

Otis, T. Measuring "quality of life" in urban areas. *Evaluation*, 1972, *1*, 35–38.

Proposed in this article is the development of a social-environmental audit system as a way of measuring the quality of life in an urban area. Quality of life is defined as encompassing such variables as job opportunities, education, public safety, citizen participation, and transportation. Four to five indicators, reflecting such categories, were selected by program staff. The potential utility of this strategy is discussed by the author.

Redick, R. W., Goldsmith, H. F., & Unger, E. L. *1970 census data used to indicate areas with different potentials for mental health and related problems.* Rockville, Md.: National Institute of Mental Health, 1971.

This paper reviews the initial stages of a project designed to evaluate efficient, low cost procedures used to provide data for effective mental health planning. The major discussion focuses on examining the dimensions of social area analysis and their sensitivity to variation in social and demographic characteristics of urban subareas. The concluding section on demographic profiles illustrates the use of 1970 census tract summary tapes in health planning for Dane County, Wisconsin.

Richard, R. *Subjective social indicators.* Chicago: National Opinion Research Center, University of Chicago, 1969.

This report is a methodologic study designed to define and measure a "social profile of target areas" by identifying and aggregating relevant variables. The term *subjective* in the title refers to measures such as attitudes, preferences, and aspirations. Such profiles have potential utility for policy makers and social-action agencies involved in program planning, program development, and evaluation research.

Rosen, B. M. *A model for estimating mental health needs using 1970 census socioeconomic data.* Rockville, Md.: National Institute of Mental Health, 1974.

Illustrated in this paper is a method for using the Mental Health Demographic Profile System as applied to Montgomery County, Maryland. Age-sex-color population pyramids are discussed as well as social and economic variables. The author concludes that the integration of the profile system with mental health utilization data can provide an adequate assessment for small area planning. Extensive tables supplement the discussion.

Rossi, D. M. Community social indicators. In A. Campbell & P. E. Converse (Eds.), *The human meaning of change.* New York: Russell Sage Foundation, 1972, pp. 87–126.

This chapter begins with an overview of the concept of community and the problems inherent in its definition and measurement. However, the major emphasis entails setting forth the variables that could be captured by the proposed social-psychological indicators. The four groupings of indicators include: orientations to localities as collectivities, the measurement of integration, relationships to central local institutions, and aspects of housing. The author also discusses strategies for chosing the appropriate model.

Sheldon, E. B., & Parke, R. Social indicators. *Science,* 1975, *188,* 693–699.

Drs. Sheldon and Parke review the development and utilization of social indicators. Their conceptual and methodologic refinement is discussed, and improvements in the data base are illustrated. The authors also examine the inclusion of social indicators in social systems models. The conclusion emphasizes the contributions of social indicators and their potential for continued impact on scientific measurement of social change.

Sheldon, E., & Moore, W. E. (Eds.). *Indicators of social change: Concepts and measurement*. New York: Russell Sage Foundation, 1968.

The authors of this volume have focused their attention on defining and measuring social change in an analytic, rather than practical, manner pointing out the complexity of change in this society. Five major topics are included in this book: (1) demographic base and shifts, (2) major structural components of society, (3) distributive features of American society, (4) aggregative features of American society, and (5) the meaning of welfare.

Shevky, E., & Bell, W. *Social area analysis: Theory, illustrative application and computational procedures*. Stanford: Stanford University Press, 1955.

Basic orientation, construct formation, and index construction for social area analysis are presented in this monograph. It demonstrates the use of this approach for the comparative study of certain social structure aspects found in American cities. Possible applications and modifications are suggested, and a social area analysis of the San Francisco Bay Region exemplifies the methodology. Computational procedures are also discussed in depth.

Stewart, R., & Poaster, L. Methods of assessing mental and physical health needs from social statistics. *Evaluation*, 1975, *2*, 67–70.

Three methods are presented that have been employed for assessing needs in the small community of Modesto, California. Visual identification, census tract identification, and variations of absolute numbers in a specific disorder are discussed in terms of their different use of social statistics. The authors note the major strengths and weaknesses inherent in each method.

Taeuber, C. (Ed.). America in the seventies: Some social indicators. *The Annals of the American Academy of Political and Social Science*, 1978, *435*.

This is a special issue of *The Annals* edited by Dr. Conrad Taeuber of Georgetown University. Included in this issue are the major findings published by the U. S. Government (*Social Indica-*

*tors,* 1976). Among the topics covered in this issue by leading social scientists are: (1) earning and spending practices; (2) population dynamics; (3) health and health care trends; (4) changing family styles; (5) crime trends; (6) educational, racial, and class relationships; and (7) the use of leisure.

Taylor, D. G., Aday, L. A., & Anderson, R. A social indicator of access to medical care. *Journal of Health and Social Behavior,* 1975, *16,* 39–49.

This investigation concentrates on the symptoms-response ratio and the related problems of under- and overutilization of services by different groups, as determined in part by access to services. The computation and reliability of the symptoms-response index are discussed in detail and applied to a national sample of the United States. The authors argue that, based on their findings, the indicator of access can be a key factor in measuring the progress of health care in attaining its goals.

Theordorson, G. A. (Ed.). *Studies in human ecology.* Evanston, Ill.: Row Peterson, 1961.

A collection of essays illustrating the major approaches to studying human ecology is presented in this book. The theory and research sections contain articles advocating and criticizing the classical position, and several essays focusing on the neoorthodox and sociocultural approaches and on social area analysis. Two other sections report on over twenty studies, both regional and cross-cultural. Also, there is one section devoted to essays on human geography.

U.S. Department of Health, Education, and Welfare. *Toward a social report.* Washington, D. C.: U.S. Government Printing Office, 1969.

This report is oriented toward the development of comprehensive social indicators that can reflect the social progress of the United States. The seven areas targeted for discussion and evaluation include health and illness, social mobility, physical environment, income and poverty, public order and safety, learning, science, and art, and participation and alienation. Questions are raised, and hypotheses are explored in an effort to refine the process of social reporting.

U.S. Bureau of the Census. *Census tract papers, series GER-40, No. 9. Social indicators for small areas.* Presented at the Conference on Small-Area Statistics, American Statistical Association, Montreal, Canada. Washington, D.C.: U.S. Government Printing Office, 1973.

A collection of five papers in this monograph covers the following topics related to the use of composite social indicators for small areas: recent developments in methodology, specific examples of applied methodology, a case study of Los Angeles using the Scientific Urban Matrix, issues in the generation and use of indicators, procedures and applications based on the Mental Health Demographic Profile System.

Wallace, H. M., Eisner, V., & Dooley, S. Availability and usefulness of selected health and socioeconomic data for community planning. *American Journal of Public Health,* 1967, *57,* 762–771.

Identified in this paper are the availability of health and social indices in San Francisco. Comparisons are made between two methods (plotting of data on maps and factor analysis), and their usefulness for identifying high-risk census tracts is determined. Findings from each of these methods tend to complement those of the other method. The most useful health and socioeconomic indices are also cited in this study.

Walton, F. What social indicators don't indicate. *Evaluation,* 1973, *1,* 79–83.

A critical appraisal of social indicators is presented in this article. Citing a specific study, Mr. Walton points out some of the conceptual and practical difficulties in using social indicators. In particular, the inherent arbitrary nature of social indicators presents a special political problem. Steps that can be taken to remedy the situation are suggested by the author.

Wennburg, J., & Gittlesohn, A. Small area variations in health care delivery. *Science,* 1973, *182,* 1102–1108.

This paper examines the variations evident among neighboring communities in Vermont based on measurement of resource input, utilization of services, and health care expenditures. The authors discuss the concept of a population-based health care system and document their position by evaluating specific policy decisions that were not supported by adequate information.

Wilcox, L. D., Brooks, R. M., Beal, G. M., & Klonglan, G. E. *Social indicators and societal monitoring: An annotated bibliography.* San Francisco: Jossey-Bass, 1972.
Included in this extensive literature search are over 1,000 separate listings, of which over 600 have been annotated. The annotated topics include: (1) definition, (2) concepts, (3) methodology, (4) policy and planning, (5) application, (6) criticism and state of the art, (7) bibliography, and (8) related subjects. The volume is of potential utility to those interested in acquiring initial knowledge and those with more specialized interests in social indicator research.

Windle, C., Rosen, R. M., Goldsmith, H. F., & Shambaugh, J. P. A demographic system for comparative assessment of "needs" for mental health services. *Evaluation,* 1975, *2,* 73–76.
This report outlines the contributions of the Mental Health Demographic Profile System in using simple data inexpensively. The authors discuss the system in terms of its inputs, outputs, and application to planning and evaluation. Figures illustrate the types of information that can be extracted by this type of data analysis.

## C. Nominal Group and Delphi Technique

Dalkey, N. G., Rourke, D. L., Lewis, R., & Snyder, D. *Studies in the quality of life.* Lexington, Mass.: Lexington Books, 1972.
This book focuses on the application of the Delphi method in studying the quality of life. Chapter two presents the rationale and procedures used to implement this approach in group decision making. Normalized estimates, error, and deviations are discussed in detail. The remaining two chapters emphasize the contributions of the Delphi method, experimentally and as applied to quality of life models.

Delbecq, A. L., & Van de Ven, A. H. A group process model for problem identification and program planning. *Journal of Applied Behavioral Science,* 1971, *7,* 466–492.

A program planning model, designed for structuring decision making in different phases of planning, is described in this article. Five phases are outlined: problem exploration, knowledge exploration, priority development, program development, and program evaluation. The situational characteristics of the group process at each phase are discussed in detail as the authors attempt to integrate small group theory (meeting formats) with community planning (reference groups).

Delbecq, A. L., Van de Ven, A. H., & Gustafson, D. H. *Group techniques for program planning: A guide to Nominal Group and Delphi processes.* Glenview, Ill.: Scott, Foresman, 1975.

This book is oriented toward human services practitioners, with "practice" being broadly defined. The first chapter introduces the reader to the need for group methods in "judgmental decision making." Chapter two reviews the research on small group decision making. Chapters three and four provide explicit and detailed guidelines for the use of the nominal group technique and the Delphi technique. The last chapter focuses on applying the nominal group technique in planning situations.

Huber, G. P., & Delbecq, A. L. Guidelines for combining the judgments of individual members in decision conferences. *Academy of Management Journal,* 1972, 6, 161–174.

This study addresses the problem of combining judgments of a number of group members into a single group judgment. Specific variables investigated include: (1) alternative response scales, (2) alternative aggregate rules for transforming individual judgments into group-representative judgments, (3) the number of group members, and (4) the accuracy of the judgments of the individual group members. The error contained in the group judgments, in general, was affected by each of these variables. Guidelines for structuring decision making are suggested.

Linstone, H. A., & Turoff, M. (Eds.). *The Delphi method.* Reading, Mass.: Addison-Wesley, 1975.

This collection of essays is divided into six major categories: philosophy, general applications, evaluation, cross-impact analysis, specialized techniques, and computers and Delphi. The edi-

tors offer a general overview of the Delphi method in the introduction, and they discuss eight basic pitfalls in a summary chapter. Many applied studies are included in this comprehensive
volume on the techniques and procedures involved in the Delphi
approach.

Van de Ven, A., & Delbecq, A. L. Nominal vs. interacting group
processes for committee decision-making effectiveness. *Academy
of Management Journal,* 1971, *14,* 204–211.

Drs. Van de Ven and Delbecq present a literature review
comparing nominal group processes with those of an interactive
approach. Topical issues focus on the relationship of group process to creative problem-solving. The implications for committee
decision making effectiveness are outlined with the authors' recommendations for the appropriate interface of these two types
of group processes.

Van de Ven, A. H., & Delbecq, A. L. The Nominal Group as a
research instrument for exploratory health studies. *American
Journal of Public Health,* 1972, *62,* 337–442.

After a brief description of problems confronting a health
services planner, the authors present a detailed description of the
nominal group process. In discussing nominal groups used in
pilot research, specific methodological difficulties are analyzed.
The advantages of the process are enumerated, particularly as
they apply to the judgmental character of health planning
efforts.

Van de Ven, A. H., & Delbecq, A. L. The effectiveness of Nominal, Delphi, and interacting group decision making processes.
*Academy of Management Journal,* 1974, *17,* 605–621.

Three alternative methods for group decision making—interacting, Nominal, and Delphi processes—are compared in this
study. The criteria used to measure the comparative effectiveness
of these strategies include the quantity of unique ideas generated
by the groups and the perceived satisfaction of groups with the
decision-making process in which the participants were involved.
In general, it is found that the nominal and Delphi groups are
equally effective, and both are clearly more effective than conventional groups.

## D. Survey

Bentz, W. D., Hollister, W. G., Edgerton, W. J., Miller, R. T., & Aponte, J. F. *Experiences in rural mental health: Surveys.* Chapel Hill: University of North Carolina Press, 1974.

Representing one of a series of booklets in *Experiences in Rural Mental Health,* this booklet deals with the assessment of rural mental health needs through the use of surveys. The extent of psychiatric disorder in a community, as well as the kinds of programs, services, and professionals that the rural communities felt were needed, were determined by a preliminary survey and an after-survey upon completion of a rural feasibility project in North Carolina. Changes in identified needs and attitudes over a five-year period are discussed in this report.

Birnbaum, Z. W., & Sirken, M. G. *Design of sample surveys to estimate the prevalence of rare diseases: Three unbiased estimates.* Rockville, Md.: National Center for Health Statistics, 1965.

The design presented was constructed to alleviate two major difficulties previously experienced in rare disease assessment, that is, large sampling and nonsampling errors. The population and sampling survey are briefly described, and three formulas are presented to estimate the number of diagnosed cases. Each formula is characterized by the amount of survey information that it utilizes.

Cannel, C. F., Fowler, F. J., & Marquis, K. H. *The influence of interviewer and respondent psychological and behavioral variables on the reporting of household interviews.* Rockville, Md.: National Center for Health Statistics, 1968.

The authors present a methodologic study designed to identify major interviewer and respondent variables related to the level of reporting health information in household settings. It describes the evaluation procedures used during observed interview situations. Hypothesized relationships between key behavior variables and psychological and demographic characteristics and actual findings are discussed in detail. Appendices provide specific information on factor loadings and index construction.

Devine R. & Falk, L. *Social surveys: A research strategy for social scientist and students.* Morristown, N.J.: General Learning Press, 1972.

This monograph is intended as a teaching tool for those interested in conducting social surveys. All phases of survey research are discussed including the underlying rationale, sampling, questionnaire construction, and interviewer selection, training, and supervision. The literature in each area is reviewed, and the authors illustrate their position with examples from their experience in integrating education with applied social research.

Dohrenwend, B. P., & Dohrenwend, B. S. The problem of validity in field studies of psychological disorder. *Journal of Abnormal Psychology,* 1965, *70,* 52–68.

An overview of problems resulting from over 25 attempts to count untreated cases of psychological disorders is presented. Issues pertaining to content and construct validity are discussed in depth with suggestions for countering typical problems that limit validity. After noting the theoretical issues in relating sociocultural factors and symptomatology, the authors propose a nomologic network to further validate the construct of psychological disorder.

Kish, L. *Survey sampling.* New York: John Wiley, 1965.

This book is designed to provide a working knowledge of practical sampling methods oriented to surveys of human populations. Detailed analyses of techniques and formulas as well as discussions of theoretical concepts constitute over half the text. The remaining sections focus on special problems and techniques, biases and nonsampling errors, and issues related to statistical inference.

Lansing, J. B., & Morgan, J. N. *Economic survey methods.* Ann Arbor, Michigan: Survey Research Center, Institute for Social Research, University of Michigan, 1971.

A detailed examination of survey methodology is contained in this book. After discussing the development and purposes of economic surveys, the authors evaluate different types of designs and illustrate them with specific studies. Sampling problems, data collection, data analysis, and financial organization and utilization are the topical areas covered in depth. Several chapters are supplemented with an extensive reference list.

Marquis, K. H., & Cannell, C. F. *Effects of some experimental interviewing techniques on reporting in health interview survey.* Rockville, Md.: National Center for Health Statistics, 1971.

The design presented in this study is based on previous research findings confirming the effects of the interviewer's behavior on the activity level of the respondent. The goal was to increase the amount and quality of reported health information. The study plan, the sample, and the differential effectiveness of various techniques are discussed in detail. The questionnaires used are included in the appendix.

Moser, C. A. *Survey methods in social investigation.* London: Heinemann, 1958.

This book begins with a discussion on the nature of social surveys, their evolution in Great Britain, their planning, and their coverage. However, its major focus is on methodology. Sampling is analyzed in detail, and data collection based on documents, observations, mail questionnaires, and interviews is discussed. Separate chapters illustrate questionnaire construction, response errors, and data analysis, interpretation, and presentation.

Robin, S. A procedure for securing returns to mail questionnaires. *Sociology and Social Research,* 1965, *50,* 24–35.

This paper describes a technique that resulted in high returns for ten independent samples. The author proposes that the difficulties, in terms of population definition and sampling procedure, posed by low rates of return can be mitigated by using the method presented. The procedures and results from the ten samples are discussed in detail.

Schwartz, R. Follow-up by phone or by mail. *Evaluation,* 1973, *1,* 25–26.

Comparisons between mail and telephone follow-up questionnaires indicate that the telephone interview yields a significantly higher rate of response (35 percent vs. 85 percent). No significant difference was found between the types of respondent (patient vs. relative). However, certain questions did elicit different responses from patients and relatives. Implications for data collection are discussed in the article.

Survey Research Center. *Interviewer's manual.* Ann Arbor, Michigan: Institute for Social Research, University of Michigan, 1976.

This manual begins with an overview of the Survey Research Center and the type of programs it conducts. Also, general information about surveys is included as an introduction. However, the major emphasis is on principles and procedures for interviewing and sampling. Questionnaires, tape-recording, nonresponses, segmented interviewing, and respondent selection are some of the topics covered. Administrative procedures are mentioned in the concluding section.

Turner, R. J., Gardner, E. A., & Higgins, A. C. Epidemiological data for mental health center planning. I. Field survey methods in social psychiatry: The problem of the lost population. *American Journal of Public Health*, 1970, *60*, 1040–1051.

Attention is called to the problem of lost populations in field surveys by the authors of this paper. In general, they find that unskilled individuals are overrepresented in lost populations. The authors suggest that both identification of the lost population and knowledge of the reason for the loss aid in estimating the degree and direction of bias in interviewed survey samples.

Webb, K., & Hatry, H. P. *Obtaining citizen feedback: The application of citizen surveys to local government.* Washington, D.C.: Urban Institute, 1973.

The booklet details the uses of citizen surveys and the dangers and pitfalls involved. The introduction provides an overview of the topic and the rationale for the report. Chapters cover survey procedures, costs and funding sources, and organization options for undertaking surveys. Several studies are cited to illustrate various applications of the survey technique. The concluding chapter lists specific recommendations for utilization.

## E. Key Informant, Community Forums, and Other Approaches

Barker, R. G. *Ecological psychology: Concepts and methods for studying the environment of human behavior.* Stanford, Calif.: Stanford University Press, 1968.

This book describes concepts, field methods, and analytical programs for investigating human behavior and its environment in real-life situations. The influence of behavior settings on human behavior is demonstrated by empirical evidence, and methods of identifying them and determining their attributes are given by Dr. Barker. A theory of the relationship between these settings and behavior is also detailed.

Barker, R. G., & Schoggen, P. *Qualities for community life.* San Francisco: Jossey-Bass, 1973.

The changes over a decade in the living conditions of two towns—one American and one English—and the consequent changes in the behavior of the inhabitants are described in this book. Of particular importance are the ways of describing and measuring the character and quality of the towns' life and living. The authors describe measuring the person-place units, referred to as behavior settings. Other innovative measures are identified in the book. All are applicable in the investigation of communities, institutions, and towns.

Buhl, J. M., Warheit, G. J., & Bell, R. A. The key informant approach to community needs assessment: A case study. *Evaluation and Program Planning,* 1978, *1,* 239–247.

Included in this paper is a description of the methods and techniques that were employed in a mailed questionnaire key informant study conducted in Jefferson County, Kentucky. Both the advantages and disadvantages of this approach to need assessment are discussed. The data collected from the key informant study is compared with findings obtained from a social indicator study of the same geographical area. Programmatic recommendations are also included in the paper.

Campbell, D. T. The informant in quantitative research. *American Journal of Sociology,* 1955, *60,* 339–342.

The study focuses on establishing the reliability of using key informants. The data is from an examination of the comparative morale of ten submarine crews where the rankings given by three offship informants are correlated with rankings anonymously given by all crew members. The techniques and specific data analysis are discussed by Dr. Campbell.

Dunham, H. W. *Community and schizophrenia: An epidemiological analysis.* Detroit: Wayne State University Press, 1965.

The essential purpose of this book is to report the findings of an intensive epidemiologic study of two subcommunities in Detroit. Previous studies are noted, and the problem of "true" incidence rates is examined. The survey is presented with many graphs and tables, and the results are discussed in terms of the relationship of social structures and schizophrenia. Theoretical and empirical implications are examined in a general summary.

Hollister, W. G., Edgerton, W. J., Bentz, W. K., Miller, F. T., & Aponte, J. F. *Experiences in rural mental health: Developing citizen participation.* Chapel Hill: University of North Carolina Press, 1974.

This pamphlet describes the development of citizen participation, through the formation of neighborhood Advisory Councils, in a rural mental health program. These councils were formed in an attempt to identify the needs and to develop programs for the rural area. Three process phases were involved in their development: (1) problem defining and priority setting, (2) discussing and studying possible solutions, and (3) recommending a program for the community to alleviate the identified problem.

MacMahan, B. Epidemiological methods. In D. W. Clark & B. MacMahan (Eds.). *Preventive medicine.* Boston: Little, Brown, 1967, pp. 81–104.

This chapter opens with a brief discussion of definitions and uses of epidemiology. The major focus, however, is on descriptive epidemiology, formulation of hypotheses, and types of analytic studies. Variables characterizing persons and places are specifically discussed, for example, ethnicity, occupation, spot maps.

Time variables are also delineated in this overview of methodologic considerations pertinent to planning epidemiologic studies.

Newbrough, J. R., & Christenfeld, R. M. *Community mental health epidemiology: Nashville. Final report of a feasibility study for a program to monitor depressed mood in the local community.* Nashville, Tennessee: Center for Community Studies, 1975.

Included in this final report is a description of the chronology, background and rationale, measurement strategies, specific plans, and results of a project to monitor depressed mood in the community. Of particular interest is the section on measurement strategies for the community (information and events system) and depressed mood, and the section on implications of the project. The latter includes community epidemiology, the assessment of community mental health program needs, and social indicators.

Richman, A. Assessing the need for psychiatric care. *Canadian Psychiatric Association Journal,* 1966, *3,* 179–187.

This essay reviews the validity of epidemiologic surveys. Problems are delineated under specific types of care, including those of general medicine and, particularly, those pertinent to psychiatric needs and treatment. The author discusses critical issues in the diagnostic process: social factors in physicians, natural history of the disorder, definitions of the impairment, and clinical insignificance of some statistically significant factors.

Seidler, J. On using informants: A technique for collecting quantitative data and controlling measurement error in organization analysis. *American Sociological Review,* 1974, *39,* 816–831.

Use of informants in organization studies is reviewed, and the history of the technique and its methodologic problems are discussed. An "instrumental theory" approach is applied to a study of religious organizations, and the outcome is described. The author particularly attends to guidelines for quantification of variables and the creation of error variables. Causal models of measurement are presented, and evaluation of data quality is proposed by relating error variables to substantive variables.

Tremblay, M. A. The key informant technique: A nonethnographic application. *American Anthropologist,* 1957, *59,* 686–701.
Actual data are used in this article to illustrate the implementation of the key informant technique in a structured but flexible research design. The author discusses in detail the stages of the process, focusing on definitions, objectives, preliminary research design, and research operations. The type of data gathered and its potential application are highlighted.

Warheit, G. J., Buhl, J. M., & Bell, R. A. A critique of social indicators analysis and key informants surveys as needs assessment methods. *Evaluation and Program Planning,* 1978, *1,* 23–30.
The practicality and utility of social indicators analysis and key informants surveys are compared in this pilot study. Social indicators analysis successfully identified different areas of need in the geographical area under study. The authors suggest that this method is a practical and valid means for assessing needs at a general level. Key informant surveys were found to be less useful. Informants were not able to identify different types of needs or their geographical distribution.

Young, R. W., & Young, R. C. Key informant reliability in rural Mexican villages. *Human Organization,* 1961, *209,* 141–148.
After a brief overview on the key informant technique the authors discuss the particulars of their study. Issues covered in detail include the criteria of reliability, the effect of the type of information asked and the level of precision required, and the consistency and stability of the informant's perspective. The summary points out the conditions that affect reliability and offers suggestions for the use of this technique.

### IV. UTILIZATION AND APPLICATION

Center for Social Research and Development. *An analysis and synthesis of needs assessment research in the field of human services.* Denver: Denver Research Institute, 1974.
Included in this report are a review and analysis of a number

of "needs assessment" efforts. Among its conclusions related to the use of need assessment data are the need for: (1) a user-based rather than an imposed design, (2) a specific program focus, (3) research conducted by an independent research team, (4) involvement by the research team with potential users, and (5) legitimacy and ability of users to change the foci of their organization.

Moore, D. N., Bloom, B. L., Gaylin, S., Pepper, M., Pettus, C., Willis, E. M., & Bahn, A. K. Data utilization for local community mental health program development. *Community Mental Health Journal*, 1967, *3*, 30–32.

This short essay outlines a systematic approach to data collection for planning and evaluating community mental health services. Issues and problems in utilizing data for local community mental health program development are identified. Specific applications are cited, and suggestions are made to bridge the gap between researchers and decision-makers.

Morrison, B. J., & Sundel, M. Development of a community assessment strategy for program evaluation in a comprehensive human service delivery system. In J. Zusman & C. Wurster (Eds.), *Program evaluation: Alcohol, drug abuse, and mental health services.* Lexington, Mass: D.C. Heath, 1975, pp. 161–170.

Ms. Morrison and Dr. Sundel report on the development of a community assessment strategy in a comprehensive human service delivery system. After describing the region, the authors identify community assessment data sources including a community assessment profile reflecting major social area analysis constructs, client data, and other data such as police statistics. The authors discuss how the data can be used in administration, prevention, outreach, consultation, community education, and treatment activities. Steps to maximize utilization of the community assessment information are also identified.

Murrell, S. A. Eight process steps for converting need assessment data into program operations. In R. A. Bell, M. Sundel, J. F. Aponte, & S. A. Murrell (Eds.), *Need assessment in health and human services: Proceedings of the Louisville National Conference.* Louisville, Kentucky, 1976, pp. 91–109.

The author first suggests criteria for a successful need assessment, which includes data being utilized in agency decisions and policies. Eight ways in which a needs assessor can promote utilization, including an "in-loop" assessment are identified. Different need assessment methods are discussed in terms of the amount of risk they pose to agencies and organizations.

Murrell, S. A. Utilization of need assessment for community decision-making. *American Journal of Community Psychology,* 1977, 5, 461–468.

Dr. Murrell describes procedures for increasing need assessment utilization and strategies for providing systematic information for community decision making. Of particular importance are the match between the information and the decision and the value context of the decision. An actual project is described to illustrate these procedures. Four general guides for utilization are also provided.

Schwab, J., Warheit, G., & Fennell, E. An epidemiologic assessment of needs and utilization of services. *Evaluation,* 1975, 2, 67–70.

The authors outline a five stage model for comprehensive evaluation research in a community mental health center. However, the major presentation focuses on an assessment of need and service utilization in Alachua County, Florida. Results are analyzed in terms of health care needs, utilization, and a comparison of needers and utilizers. Reliability and validity of self-report data are also discussed.

## V. EXAMPLES OF NEED ASSESSMENTS

Carr, W., & Wolfe, S. Unmet needs as sociomedical indicators. *International Journal of Health Services,* 1976, 6, 417–430.

The authors argue for comprehensive health programs in discussing the Meharry Medical College Study of Unmet Needs.

Definitions of unmet needs are discussed, particularly as they affect measures of program outcome. The limitations of various approaches to measuring unmet needs are explored in terms of the more comprehensive Meharry methodology. The concluding remarks about the significance and application of this approach offer suggestions for further research.

Mellan, W. A., & Bell, R. A. *Southern health and family life studies (Vol. III). Outcome appraisals studies: Continuity of care.* Gainesville, Fla.: Florida Mental Health Evaluation Consortium, 1974.

This volume is one of a series from the Florida Mental Health Evaluation Consortium. Included in this mongraph are a description of the comprehensive evaluation model already cited (Bell & Mellan, 1974), and a continuity of care instrument developed by this group. A general description of the instrument, reason for selection, its basic methodology, and findings and modifications concerning its overall reliability, practicality, and utility are included in this report.

Pasamanick, B., Roberts, D., Lemkau, P. V., Krueger, D. A survey of mental disease in an urban population: Prevalence by race and income. In F. Reissman, J. Cohen, & A. Pearl (Eds.), *Mental health of the poor.* New York: Free Press, 1966, pp. 39–48.

This report describes the first two phases of a study designed to estimate the prevalence of chronic disorder and the needs for care in Baltimore. The clinical evaluations of a subsample chosen from a household canvas are discussed in detail. Implications in terms of race and income as related to differences in types of chronic illness are emphasized.

Schwab, J. J., Bell, R. A., Warheit, G. J., & Schwab, R. B. *Social order and mental health.* New York: Brunner/Mazel, 1978.

This is a major study of mental health risk in a North Central Florida county. The primary objective was to assess the number of persons in this county at risk for social psychiatric impairment and to identify possible associated sociocultural factors. Particular attention is directed to the chapter on "Health Needs and Utilization of Services" and to the chapter on the "Perception of Social Change and Social Psychiatric Change."

## VI. RELATED READINGS

Bloom, B. L. *Changing patterns of psychiatric care.* New York: Human Sciences Press, 1975.

The major focus of this book is the evaluation of the consequences resulting from changes in the mental health service delivery system between 1960 and 1970. The first section provides an overview of psychopathology as a community problem and the methodologies employed to assess it. However, the essence of the changing patterns is exemplified by a reevaluation after a decade of service delivery in Pueblo County, Colorado. Subsequent sections illuminate the pattern of psychiatric care in 1970 and discuss the importance of service statistics and epidemiology.

Broskowski, A., Attkisson, C. C., Tuller, I. R., & Berk, J. H. *Human services program evaluation: An edited bibliography of key references.* Milwaukee, Wisconsin: V-U Publishing Co., 1975.

Included in this edited bibliography are references that cover the following: (1) basic summaries or syntheses of a wide range of issues, techniques, and findings; (2) organizational theory; (3) national strategy-policy research; (4) general research methodologies; (5) management information systems; (6) need assessments; (7) standards, regulations, and monitoring; (8) cost-outcome and cost-benefit analysis; (9) evaluation of training; (10) utilization-implementation; (11) confidentiality; (12) applied case studies; and (13) other bibliographies and general sources.

Coursey, R. D., Specter, G. A., Murrell, S. A., & Hunt, B. (Eds.). *Program evaluation for mental health: Methods, strategies, and participants.* New York: Grune & Stratton, 1977.

This is a practical book that focuses on setting up and running evaluation programs for real-life mental health service systems. It is divided into four major sections: (1) methods of program evaluation, (2) strategies for program evaluation, (3) participants in program evaluation, and (4) further resources. These sections summarize the current literature and provide both conceptual and practical knowledge for individuals involved in or wishing to plan and carry out program evaluations.

Demone, H. W., & Harshbarger, D. *A handbook of human service organizations.* New York: Behavioral Publications, 1974.

This volume is divided into seven major sections: (1) introduction, (2) environmental forces acting on and reacting to human service organizations, (3) central concerns of human service organizations, (4) roles and role problems, (5) management and planning tactics and strategies, (6) assessing the outcomes of administration and planning strategies, and (7) perspectives for the future. Particular attention is directed to the second section that deals with the surrounding environment, social systems, and changing subsystems.

Dohrenwend, B. S., & Dohrenwend, B. P. *Stressful life events: Their nature and effects.* New York: John Wiley, 1974.

This collection of essays provides an extensive review of research related to stressful life events. Four major sections discuss the concomitants of physical illness, clinical research on physical and psychiatric disorder, community research on psychiatric symptomatology, and methodological research on stressful life events. Critical issues are examined, and future directions for research are proposed. A summary chapter defines the nature of the role that stressful life events play in the etiology of somatic psychiatric disorders.

Langner, T. S., & Michael, S. T. *Life stress and mental health: The Midtown Manhattan Study* (Vol. II). Glencoe, Ill.: Free Press, 1963.

The first seven chapters of this classic study describe the conceptual and analytical framework, the research methods, the system of mental health ratios used, the community setting, the problems of interpretation, and the isolation of stress factors. The remaining nine chapters focus upon interpreting the actual data, including an examination of plausible hypotheses to explain the results. Various interrelationships among childhood and adult experiences, as they relate to stress, are explored in specific chapters.

Leighton, A. H. *My name is legion.* New York: Basic Books, 1959.

This is the classic Stirling County study of psychiatric disorder and the sociocultural environment that spanned 10 years from pilot inception to data presentation. Dr. Leighton describes the major goals as discovering the types of associations between disorder and environment, defining targets for more complex studies, and elucidating the problems inherent in attacking the targets. The discussion covers three areas: psychiatric disorders, psychiatric disorders and sociocultural factors, and the plan for research.

Levy, L., & Rowitz, L. *The ecology of mental disorder.* New York: Behavioral Publications, 1973.

The study presented was designed to identify ecologic characteristics of communities which produced different rates of psychiatric casualties in Chicago. The authors review the literature and outline their methodology before discussing the specific findings. Focal topics include demographic characteristics, spatial distribution, ecological analysis, and ecological attributes of high and low rates for first admission and utilization.

Mikawa, J. K. Evaluations in community mental health. In P. McReynolds (Ed.), *Advances in psychological assessment* (Vol. 3). San Francisco: Jossey-Bass, 1975, pp. 389–432.

This general commentary reviews major contributions of need assessments, outcome evaluations, and management information systems. Well-known studies and proponents of various approaches are discussed. The author explores the issues raised by different methodologies and concludes by outlining what he considers to be the major problems and the most neglected areas in evaluating community mental health.

Miller, J. G. *Living systems.* New York: McGraw-Hill, 1978.

This book presents an integrated, multidisciplinary analysis of the nature of all biologic and social systems which, according to Dr. Miller, are organized into seven hierarchical levels. Detailed analyses of the major aspects and characteristics of these levels are presented, and multiple variables, as well as practical indicators for measuring change, are identified.

Srole, L., Langner, T. S., Michael, S. T., Opler, M. K., & Rennie, T. A. *Mental health in the metropolis.* New York: McGraw-Hill, 1962.

This is the original report on the classic Midtown Manhattan Study. The goals and methodology are discussed at length, and the target community is described in terms of population distillates and psychosocial climate. However, the major position of the book is devoted to the presentation and interpretation of the findings related to mental health composition and psychiatric care in Midtown Manhattan. Ethnicity, age, sex, marital status, religion, and socioeconomic status are some of the variables discussed. The concluding commentary emphasizes the impact of the study on the relationships between community and mental health, both at theoretical and applied levels.

# INDEX